A Practic[illegible]de to Wo[illegible]ing with Depression

A cognitive behavioural approach for mental health workers

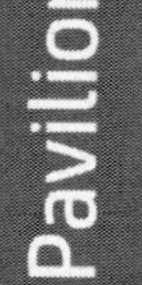

Michael O'Sullivan, Samantha Watson and Brendan Butler

A Practical Guide to Working with Depression

A cognitive behavioural approach for mental health workers

Published by:
Pavilion Publishing and Media Ltd
Rayford House
School Road
Hove BN3 5HX
UK

Tel: 01273 434 943
Fax: 01273 227 308

First published 2017

A catalogue record for this book is available from the British Library.

ISBN: 978-1-910366-90-5

Pavilion is the leading publisher and provider of professional development products and services for workers in the health, social care, education and community safety sectors. We believe that everyone has the right to fulfil their potential and we strive to supply products and services that help raise standards, promote best practices and support continuing professional development.

Authors: Michael O'Sullivan, Samantha Watson and Brendan Butler on behalf of Derbyshire Healthcare Foundation Trust

Editor: Ruth Chalmers, Pavilion Publishing and Media Ltd

Cover design: Emma Dawe, Pavilion Publishing and Media Ltd

Page layout and typesetting: Emma Dawe, Pavilion Publishing and Media Ltd

Printing: CMP Digital Print Solutions

Contents

About the authors iv

Introduction 1

Chapter 1: Where to start 3

Chapter 2: The extent of the problems 15

Chapter 3: Formulation – the links between thoughts, feelings, physical sensations and behaviours in depression 27

Chapter 4: Making sense of depression – thinking 31

Chapter 5: Making sense of depression – activity 49

Chapter 6: The therapeutic relationship 63

Chapter 7: Maintaining progress 69

About the authors

All three authors work for Derbyshire Healthcare Foundation Trust.

Michael O'Sullivan is a registered mental health nurse and a social worker. He has worked as a compassionate mind therapist for three years. He has a postgraduate diploma in cognitive behavioural psychotherapy and is registered with the British Association for Behavioural and Cognitive Psychotherapies. He is also qualified in cognitive analytic therapy.

Samantha Watson has been a registered mental health nurse since 1997. She completed the intensive dialectical behavioural therapy (DBT) training with the British Isles DBT Team, works as a mindfulness-based cognitive therapist and also has a postgraduate diploma in cognitive behavioural psychotherapy. She has been working with a compassion-focused approach since 2006. Samantha is also trained in the delivery of eye movement desensitisation and reprocessing (EMDR).

Brendan Butler is a registered mental health nurse and a social worker. He has worked as a mental health therapist for 15 years and has extensive experience in compassion-based CBT delivered in both a group and individual context. He has a degree in human psychology, a postgraduate diploma in cognitive behavioural psychotherapy and is trained in behavioural family therapy. Brendan has received training in mindfulness-based cognitive therapy.

Acknowledgement

The authors would like to thank Kim Howe for her assistance with the Qualifications Credit Framework Learning Outcomes.

Introduction

This manual is a guide for mental health workers who are relatively new to the model of cognitive behavioural therapy (CBT) in depression and who wish to use some of its techniques in their work.

The settings that this book may be useful for will range from the statutory to the non-statutory sector. Whether the worker is part of a team providing care or is working on their own, it is envisaged that they will be working on a one-to-one basis with the client. It will therefore be helpful for a range of mental health staff from community psychiatric nurses to student nurses or social workers. Because there will potentially be many different types of worker using this book we will refer throughout to the person working with the client with depression as the 'worker'. There are also of course many terms by which we describe people who use mental health services. These can range from service users to patient to client. In writing this book we have used the term 'clients'. The book contains transcripts of real life examples of work undertaken by the authors as a way of putting some of the ideas behind the manual into practice.

This manual will be useful for workers who are providing a service for clients who are depressed. The order of the chapters follows a pathway from the point when the client enters the mental health service to the point of departure, when they might leave the service. Chapter 1 looks at how motivated the client is to change. As we will explore in the book, recovery from depression involves taking a risk. Knowing how far clients are motivated to 'take that risk' is important. Chapter 2 provides an overview of depression and how it is understood within the framework of cognitive behavioural therapy. Chapter 3 develops this understanding and looks at how depression reflects the individual circumstances of the client. Chapters 4 and 5 focus on some of the tools for working with depression. Mental health workers need to be mindful of their relationship with clients with depression and the impact that this can have on their work. This is the focus of Chapter 6. Chapter 7 looks at how clients can manage their depression and maintain progress.

Each of the chapters will provide learning outcomes linked to units from the Level 2 and 3 Health and Social Care Diploma (formerly NVQ 2 & 3) in the Qualifications and Credit Framework (QCF). Because of this, the worker will need to record their work and their reflections in a journal which can be used as evidence. In using the manual, we will be asking the worker to make notes about the work that they undertake with clients. As these notes will constitute a 'medical record' any references to individual clients must be anonymous. Some of the handouts and exercises will be completed by clients. It will therefore be important for workers to ensure that clients have a folder for containing any paperwork. Any work undertaken must be consistent with the local policies of the employing organisation and national policies such as the Care Programme Approach.

Experience tells us that the reality of the client's journey is never this neat. In using this manual the worker needs to check who else may be involved with the client in order to make sure that the approach used is consistent. Most settings where CBT services exist will be in the NHS. For workers who are not in the NHS it will be helpful for them to familiarise themselves with existing CBT services. If the client is receiving CBT from a therapist then the worker will need to make sure that any work they carry out with them is consistent with the work of the therapist.

Please note: all handouts are available to download from the Pavilion website, at: https://www.pavpub.com/downloads-for-practical-guide-to-working-with-depression/

Chapter 1: Where to start

Learning outcomes

By the end of the chapter you will:

- be able to assess the client's motivation to work on change
- be aware of the potential barriers to change.

QCF units

Health and Social Care Diploma Level 2

- Unit 1: Introduction to communication in health and social care or children and young peoples' services. Learning outcomes 3.1, 3.2, 3.3, 3.4 and 4.2.

Health and Social Care Diploma Level 3

- Unit SHC 31: Promote communication in health, social care or children's and young people's settings. Learning outcomes 1, 2, 3 and 4.
- Unit SHC 33: Promote equality and inclusion in health, social care or children's and young people's settings. Learning outcomes 1, 2 and 3.

The background to this chapter is based on the ideas behind 'motivational interviewing' (Miller & Rollnick, 1991). Motivational interviewing is a set of techniques based on situations where a client believes that they need to change but feels that making the decision and the process of change will be a tough one. For the client, the perceived difficulty of the decision means that there is ambivalence about change. Throughout therapy, clients will always be in the process of weighing up the advantages and disadvantages of change because any change for the better will involve them stepping outside of their comfort zone. The theory of motivational interviewing began as an approach for working with substance abuse. However, its effectiveness has meant that it is now incorporated into a wide number of areas. As it is about finding out how motivated a client might be about change, it is in essence a cognitive approach. Motivation can be summed up by the expression 'being ready, willing and able'.

Change is not easy. There is 'safety' in depression. Recovery from depression involves someone coming out of a comfort zone and therefore entails some kind of risk. Before looking at how this might apply in your work with clients we will look at five of the principles behind the approach.

1. **Don't tell clients what they 'should' do**
   The reasons for this are straightforward in that giving advice often does not work. The more clients are able to own their decisions and the less they have to rely on other professionals, the more empowered they will become. If this rule were to be broken, it would be in the area of practical advice, for example signposting someone to the Citizen's Advice Bureau, if they need support with benefits.

2. **Active listening**
   This is very important. It is a fundamental part of most counselling courses. Again the reasons are straightforward. If you don't listen to someone it is unlikely that you will engage with them and if this happens it is even more unlikely that they will change.

3. **Client led**
   Let the client tell you they need to change. A sense of control is important in depression. The client needs to feel this. Other people such as family, other professionals or you yourself may want them to change. However, they themselves have to be willing to change for therapy to work.

4. **Ambivalence**
   Recognise ambivalence. As we have mentioned, depression can feel 'safe' while change can be risky. You can tackle ambivalence at this stage of your relationship with a client but it is likely to be a feature to some degree throughout the relationship. The perceived risks of change can be as significant as the benefits. If there are problems, then it is important to recognise ambivalence and work with it; this is more helpful than labelling the client as difficult or resistant.

5. **Ability**
   Clients need to have a belief that they can change. Their confidence may be low, but if they feel that change is difficult but not impossible then any therapy has a higher chance of success. The following sections take these ideas one step forward, and outline some of the areas that you can work on in starting the change process.

Communication skills in engagement

Reflection

Your relationship with the client is the cornerstone of your work. The idea that is fundamental to the relationship is empathy (Beck *et al*, 1979). Being empathic is very important, however it is one thing to believe that you as a worker are empathic, the client needs to actually see you as empathic. Your empathy needs to be recognised by them. There are ways of talking which can help to develop empathy. Look at the following example. Reflecting emotions back to a client can act as a way of communicating empathy.

Client: *'I'm scared of showing my emotions.'*

Worker: *'So you're afraid of showing your feelings?'*

Summaries

For clients, interactions with mental health professionals can sometimes be intimidating. There is a lot of information to take on board and this can be a problem, particularly given that a feature of depression can be difficulties in concentration. Not being able to concentrate, and the 'shame' of disclosing this to the worker through fear of looking stupid, may mean that much of what is talked about is simply not understood. This can be made worse if workers do not watch their use of jargon. You can respond to this through offering small summaries and checking with the client whether it is correct and if anything has been left out.

Worker: *'So far we've talked about the difficulties that you experience in your average day, and when those problems first begun. Does that make sense and is there anything we've left out?'*

Open questions

A standard technique in many counselling courses involves using open questions. These are questions which in essence demand more than one word answers. Examples might include:

'What are the reasons for saying that?'

'How did you respond to that situation?'

The rationale for open questions is that they encourage people to talk. Direct questions which require one word answers such as, 'Do you like your job?' will have their place, but if you use too many of them it can sound too much like an interrogation.

Noticing inconsistency

Starting therapy will be about seeing where there may be conflicts between goals. Look at the following short case example.

Rebecca was depressed because she had grown up in a family where she was constantly being criticised for her supposed defects. Her family criticised her for being 'soft in the head'. She was able to deal with this for many years because her mother supported her. When her mother died she felt alone. She wanted to live as independent a life as possible and follow her dreams of going to university and studying medicine. However, her family said that she was betraying them by having ideas above her station.

Rebecca had two options. One was to feel included and loved by her family at the cost of being independent. The other was to live as independent a life as possible and risk the possibility of being rejected by her family and being alone. She was unable to resolve this conflict and became depressed. Change can, as we see below, be about a conflict between two ways of looking at the world.

Rebecca: *'I used to really push myself to get to where I wanted to get to but the family would still tell me I was stupid. Then it got worse. They began to give me a guilt trip by saying that going to university was betraying them, and that I was having ideas above my station* [becomes tearful]. *I don't know what to do.'*

Worker: *'This sounds like an area of real conflict. You want to study medicine but you also want to be accepted by your family. It sounds like both goals are going in different directions.'*

The subject of skills such as open questions has been introduced in this section. They will, however, be important to use throughout your contact with clients with depression. Consider revisiting this section when looking at the exercises in later chapters of this manual.

In the next section there is a series of exercises, which look at each of the above areas. You will need to use a notebook for these exercises. You will also need a second notebook as a reflective journal. This will be used to record your development as you progress through the manual. You will need to share the contents of both books in your supervision sessions with either your mentor or supervisor.

Exercise 1.1: Communication skills in engagement

Over the next week, monitor your work with clients using the table in Handout 1.1. Reflect on the situation afterwards. How far did it seem to help develop your relationship with that person?

Reflection

Try to practise some of these techniques discussed and make some notes of this in your journal. Discuss what your experience was in using these techniques with either your supervisor or manager. Think about how helpful these approaches are, and think about what more you might need to know about using them.

Working with ambivalence (1)

As a worker, your role will be to help the client weigh up the advantages and disadvantages of change. As we mentioned before, there is a security in depression and change involves risk. For yourselves as workers it will be important to gauge whether the client is willing and able to take the 'risk' of change. Take a look at Exercise 1.2 below (see Handout 1.2).

Exercise 1.2: Working with ambivalence (1)

Talk to the client about the importance of change. Ask them 'how important is it to change?'. Ask them to rate this level of importance on a scale of 1-10 with 1 as not important at all and 10 as the most important thing.

Having done this ask the client about the advantages and disadvantages of remaining the same and the advantages/disadvantages of change.

Reflection

In assessing the client's readiness to work on their depression, scaling questions are important because they focus the conversation on what is happening in the here and now. In using the above scale, it will then be natural to ask the question of what is 'blocking' the change from happening.

Make a note of any responses to this question in your journal. If you did use this technique, how successful or unsuccessful was it? If the client was able to give an answer on a scale, did it seem to have any effect?

Working with ambivalence (2)

Given the perceived risk of change, it is likely that there will be resistance from the client. There is a lot of shame and stigma associated with depression. Earlier in this chapter we talked about the ambivalence of change. Clients with depression can feel shame and guilt for not being able to cope. If they then feel that they are going to have to talk about such issues, then some resistance is to be expected. It will be important to consider how this might show itself.

Possible signs might include arguing, interrupting or denying. As a worker, it is ok to begin to talk about this without actually telling the client what they should do, for example, 'Can we talk about the antidepressants now?'.

In working with ambivalence, your self-awareness in your work role is important. This will be discussed in more detail in Chapter 6. However, be aware that if the client does disagree or argue with you the natural tendency will be to argue back or to just avoid the topic. Be aware of when this happens. The idea here will be to side step the argument and develop a 'conversation' with the client about their depression. It will be helpful to re-read the five principles mentioned earlier and recognise the importance of not confronting, using empathy and recognising that ambivalence is normal.

Exercise 1.3: Working with ambivalence (2)

Look at the feedback from Exercise 1.2, and fill out the table in Handout 1.3. Identify any situations where the client appeared to be arguing, denying or interrupting. Reflect on each situation and ask yourself how far you were following the five principles outlined above.

Reflection

Record your findings in your journal. It may be that there are no examples you can think of. If this is the case, identify what you were doing. Were the majority of the situations ones which did not focus on depression but were concerned with other problems, such as benefits? If the situations were ones in which you were talking with the client about depression, what were you doing 'right'? Record any thoughts you have into your reflective journal and use them in any feedback sessions with either your mentor or supervisor.

Self-efficacy

When you are clearer about their commitment to change you need to support their self-efficacy. This reflects the last of the five principles (ability) and is about the 'able' part of 'ready, willing and able'. If they don't feel able they may not have the confidence to change. Change may be difficult but if the client feels 'able' to change as well as being ready and willing, then they may be able to do the necessary work.

Building self-efficacy will be used throughout your work with them. At this point in the relationship it is important to make a start.

Exercise 1.4: Self-efficacy

Ask the client to identify: 1) when the problem is at its height, 2) when the problem is less, and 3) when there is no problem.

The reasons for these questions are straightforward. There will be times when the client is feeling competent and able in what they are doing. Be careful to distinguish the difference between actions which appear to provide temporary relief and those which provide something more permanent. Look at the following example.

Worker: *'So if you feel anxious you usually cope by going to bed and avoiding contact with the outside world. How does that work?'*

Client: *'I feel less anxious.'*

Worker: *'Does it fix things permanently?'*

Client: *'It takes a bad feeling away for a bit but then I just become more depressed.'*

Now compare the above statement with this example.

Worker: *'So when you feel anxious you go to the gym and run for 40 minutes on the treadmill – how does that work?'*

Client: *'I get something from it: I feel better.'*

Make a record in your reflective journal about what provides more permanent improvements in the client's mood.

The idea of coping with something which provides 'short-term' relief, but does little to help the problem, occurs later on in this manual as does the idea that activities (such as going to the gym) are linked with an improvement in mood.

Goal setting

Exercise 1.4 should have given you an idea of the ways that depression has had an impact on the client. The previous exercises will have given you a sense of what the barriers are for that client in overcoming their depression. In understanding depression it is helpful to recognise that each problem has a solution that is 'in built'.

The following section looks at goals. One thing to remember, however, is that goals need to be flexible. As your work with the client progresses, the goals may change in the light of new information (Neenan & Dryden, 2002).

Exercise 1.5: Goal setting

Revisit the change scaling question from Exercise 1.2. Ask the client what they would like to change, and how, if there were no barriers to this. What they would be doing, who they would be with/not with, how they would look if they were being recorded on a video camera. Ask them to provide as much detail as possible, and encourage them to focus on body posture, vocal tone, as well as the content of what they are saying (not other physical attributes). After they have provided this description, ask them how they feel emotionally having provided this description. Then ask them how they would feel if they could act in this way in real life. Work with them on summarising this picture of what they would be like when they are well. In the final chapter of this book we will return to goal setting.

Reflection

Because mood states such as sadness are part of the human condition, knowing when a depression ends may not be clear cut. People can have 'good and bad' days when they are depressed and when they are well.

Finding out what makes things better and/or worse from clients using Exercise 1.4 can begin to develop their self-efficacy and the belief that change is possible. Exercise 1.5 starts them thinking about what mental wellness may look like to them – their own 'signature' of good mental health.

If you were able to identify the goals of the client, make a note in your reflective journal and describe the skills you were using. What did you think helped in the interaction?

Conclusion

It goes without saying that thinking is important in cognitive therapy. The problem is more often than not the client's 'perception' of their situation, rather than the situation itself. For some, isolation may not necessarily be a problem while for others it is. One client may be depressed because they perceive that their life is meaningless. Another client may be able to accept this. At the end of this section, you should be clearer about how willing the client is to work on their depression. It may be that they have considered the risks and feel too scared to change. It is important to remember that not being ready to work on change is not a failure. As mentioned earlier, depression still has a stigma – people can be ashamed of their mental health issues and the decision to change can be tough. Other interventions such as medication also exist. Psychological therapies like CBT are but one approach within mental health. However, assuming that the client is ready to change, let's move onto the next chapter.

References

Beck AT, Rush AJ, Shaw BF & Emery G (1979) *Cognitive Therapy of Depression*. New York: Guilford Press.

Miller WR & Rollnick S (1991) *Motivational Interviewing: Preparing people to change addictive behaviour.* New York: Guildford Press.

Neenan M & Dryden W (2002) *Life Coaching: A cognitive behavioural approach*. Hove: Routledge.

Handout 1.1

Exercise 1.1: Communication skills in engagement

Technique	Situation
Reflection	
Summaries	
Open questions	
Noticing discrepancies	

Handout 1.2

Exercise 1.2: Working with ambivalence (1)

Talk to the client about the importance of change. Ask them 'how important is it to change?' Ask them to rate this level of importance on a scale of 1-10 with 1 as not important at all and 10 as the most important thing.

1: No importance **10: Most important**

Having done this, ask the client about the advantages and disadvantages of remaining the same and the advantages/disadvantages of change.

Notes

Handout 1.3

Exercise 1.3: Working with ambivalence (2)

Look at the results from Exercise 1.2 and fill out the following table. Identify any situations where the client appeared to be arguing, denying or interrupting. Reflect on each situation and ask yourself how far you were following the five principles outlined above.

Examples of resistance	Situation
Arguing	
Denying	
Interrupting	

Chapter 2: The extent of the problems

Learning outcomes

By the end of this chapter you will:

- have an overview understanding of the causes and presentation of clinical depression
- have an overview understanding of the differences between depression and other mental health problems and how they overlap
- be able to apply this understanding to the work undertaken with clients.

QCF units

Health and Social Care Diploma Level 3

- Unit CMH 301: Understand mental well-being and mental health promotion. Learning outcomes 1 and 2 .

What is depression?

Before starting, it will be useful to know some facts and figures relating to depression. Evidence from six European countries found that 17% of the population recorded had some experience with depression in the last six months. Major depression accounts for 6.9% of this.

The number of people experiencing depression in recent years has risen and does not account for those who do not visit their GP and report their symptoms. The number of depressed people who do not seek mental health services is greater than the number that does so. Only 12% see a specialist for their problem, the risk of suicide increases with each new episode and each new episode of depression increases the likelihood of a relapse in the future. Depression also rarely occurs on its own and the most likely additional problem is anxiety. In fact, anxiety and depression usually go hand in hand and if you are depressed you are also more likely to experience an anxiety disorder than if not depressed and vice versa (Beck *et al*, 1979).

People suffering from depression have five times more days absent from work than others, and depression is one of the most common causes of extended absence in white collar workers. The World Health Organization has projected that by 2020 depression will be the disease to impose the second largest economic burden of ill health worldwide (World Bank, 1993).

There are differences between acute and chronic depression and clients with persistent (chronic) depression often feel hopeless and demoralised. The impact of major depression not only affects the individual sufferer but also their partners, family and friends. In fact, the impact is greater than many other conditions with the exception of heart disease. Persistent depression has drastic effects on the individual and their ability to carry out their role in society. Although low self-esteem can be seen as a vulnerability factor or antecedent to depression, the longer the depression goes on the more likely it is to lower self-esteem even further. This can result in changes in personality and an increase in dependency. When we begin to think of depression in this way, we begin to understand the differences between ordinary sadness and depression as a mental health problem. Older clients are more vulnerable to depression, with more women experiencing the condition than men. People become more likely to develop depression when they experience negative life events such as marital problems or redundancy. Clinical depression, sometimes known as major depression, consists of a combination of elements rather than a single feature. Clinical depression differs from sadness in that it is severe enough to interfere with a person's ability to function on a day-to-day basis. In order to diagnose depression, a psychiatrist will use the framework outlined in the Diagnostic and Statistical Manual Volume 5 (DSM -5). The DSM-5 lists five different types of depression (American Psychiatric Association, 2013). For the purposes of this manual we will be considering more severe depression. The areas to take into account when thinking of depression are listed below.

Symptoms of depression

1. **Depressed mood –** this means depressed for most of the day, nearly every day, as indicated by subjective report (i.e. what the individual client says) or observation by other people – family, friends or other professionals.
2. **Markedly diminished interest or pleasure –** the client experiences a loss of interest and pleasure in almost all activities most of the day, nearly every day.
3. **Physical symptoms –** this could be significant weight loss when not dieting, or weight gain. It might also include a decrease or increase in appetite nearly every day.
4. **Sleep –** the client may experience insomnia or excess sleep most days.
5. **Psychomotor agitation or retardation –** this term describes subjective feelings of restlessness or being slowed down. This may also be observed by others – family, friends or other professionals.
6. **Fatigue or loss of energy –** the client experiences these physical symptoms nearly every day.
7. **Thoughts about being worthless and feelings of excessive or inappropriate guilt –** the client with clinical depression can experience these thoughts and feelings nearly every day.

8. **Concentration** – the client's ability to think or concentrate is affected. They may feel unable to make a decision (again, this can be either subjective or observed by others).

9. **Recurrent thoughts of death** – this may include frequent ideas about suicide. This does not necessarily mean that they have a plan or intention to commit suicide.

A client might not experience all of these features. For a diagnosis to be confirmed there usually needs to be five or more of the above present. As well as severity, we also think of duration. The symptoms should have been present over at least a two-week period. It should also at some level reflect a significant change from how the client was previously.

Recovery from depression

Research suggests that at least 50% of people who recover from their first episode of depression will have at least one more episode (Kupfer, 1991). Clients who have recovered from depression more than once are more vulnerable to relapsing into depression again (Judd, 1997). Clients who have recovered from a first episode are at an important crossroads in their lives. There is a probability that they will become depressed again. Recovering from depression and staying well is an important element of CBT and will be revisited in the final chapter on relapse management in this manual. We will now consider vulnerability in more detail.

Vulnerability

There are several factors that may make someone more vulnerable to depression as a clinical condition. There are three areas to look at.

1. Genetics

There is a genetic aspect to depression. If the client has a parent or close family relative who has suffered from depression they may be more likely to develop depression. It is said that clients with a close relative who has experienced depression are one and a half to three times more likely to experience depression than those who do not. How far this is important in comparison to the environment that clients grow up in is difficult to assess. Some studies indicate that 40% is down to genetics and 60% to environmental factors (Kendler *et al*, 1999).

2. Changes in the brain

What happens in the brain with depression is still relatively unknown. What we do know is that neurotransmitter function is disrupted. Neurotransmitters are chemicals in the brain, which carry signals from one part to the other. The three important neurotransmitters that affect mood are serotonin, noradrenalin and dopamine. Antidepressant medication will affect these neurotransmitters.

3. Early life experiences

People develop a vulnerability to depression. This can come with early life experiences. If people are exposed to trauma, abuse or neglect when younger they can become more vulnerable to depression when they reach adulthood. When thinking about depression it is important to recognise how these aspects of life can affect the way we look at the world. The social and economic factors we experienced, our relationships with our brothers and sisters and peers all play an important part in the development of our beliefs. These experiences leave us with what we call 'core beliefs'.

Core beliefs

Core beliefs are pervasive inflexible beliefs that we develop and that relate to the way we view ourselves, the world and the future. For people with depression they will invariably be negative.

'I am worthless, I am inadequate.'

These beliefs will also extend to other people and the world.

'Other people are better than me.'

'Other people will let me down.'

'The world is a dangerous place.'

We will also hold beliefs about our future.

'I will always be like this, my future is bleak.'

These beliefs are developed in early childhood and can make us vulnerable to developing depression in the future. These can be explained by using the cognitive model of depression as developed by Beck *et al* (1979). An example of this model, attributed to Beck, is given in Figure 2.1.

Due to the impact these beliefs have on our mood if we are aware of them all the time, we go on to develop intermediate beliefs (rules or assumptions) that we will call 'rules for living'. These rules allow us to function on a day-to-day basis. They are important in depression because they protect us from these core beliefs. Core beliefs such as 'I'm a failure' are at the heart of depression. Implementing a rule such as 'I should always be useful' can protect us from this core belief. A person may therefore protect themselves from their depression by proving that they are useful through working all of the time. This works until there is a 'critical life event' such as redundancy, which then triggers negative automatic thoughts leading to symptoms of depression.

Figure 2.1 **Beckian Depression Model**

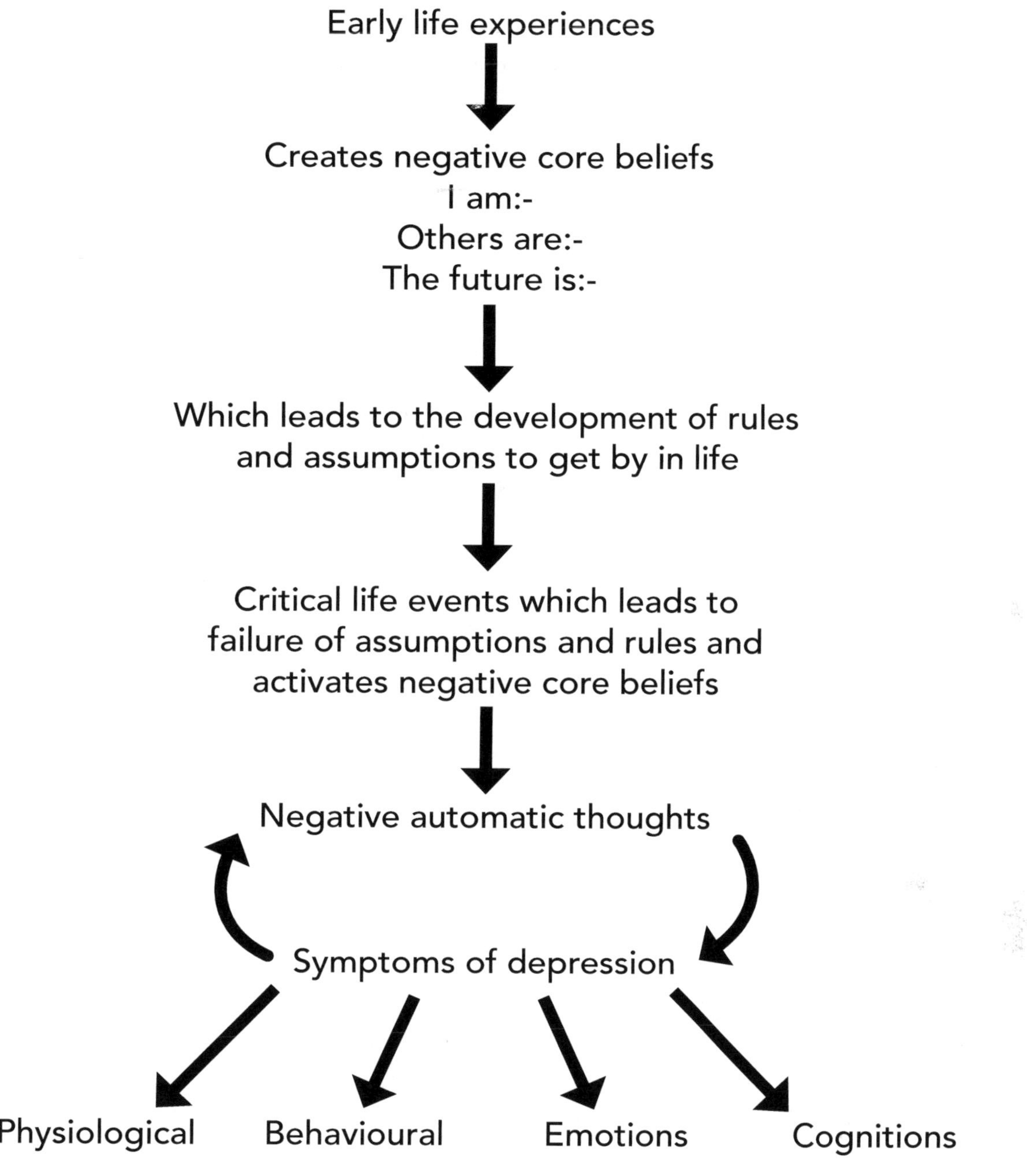

In the example in Figure 2.2, the client has developed a rule for living in response to a core belief of being worthless. In an attempt to feel valued they try to please everyone, often at the expense of their own needs. We can see the logic of this approach.

However, trying to please everyone is impossible. It may work initially but the person will start to feel used or treated like a 'doormat'. Because of their core belief they may end up thinking that somehow it is their fault because of their worthlessness. They therefore try harder. This realisation may result in the onset of depression as the rule is no longer valid. When the rule breaks down, the client will then get in touch with their negative core beliefs. Once these beliefs are activated this will affect their thinking and their mood will become lower. Once their mood becomes low they will be more likely to become more critical of themselves. This will in turn lower their mood and create a vicious circle.

Figure 2.2

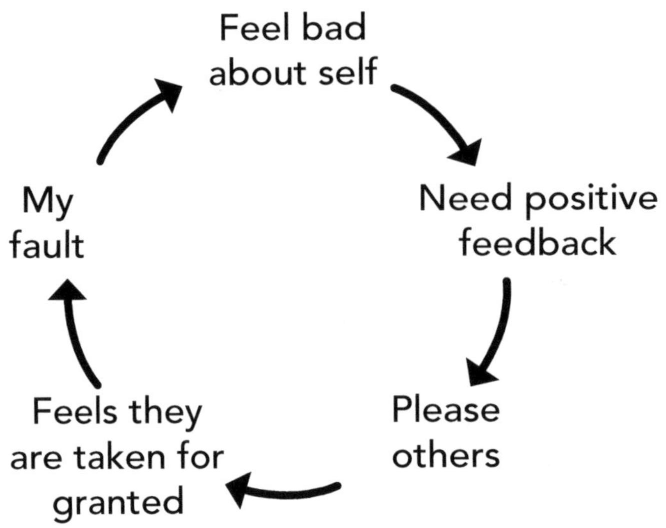

Feel bad about self → Need positive feedback → Please others → Feels they are taken for granted → My fault → Feel bad about self

We will look further at this model later on in the manual and will talk about these beliefs in more detail in Chapter 4. However, at this stage it is worth mentioning the role that medication plays in treating depression.

Medication

Treatment for depression centres on the emotional and biological effects of the disorder. Medication may be aimed at these specific symptoms. More often than not, these will be antidepressants. Some clients respond well to medication while others will not.

In the course of your work you may find that clients may talk about having their medication changed. The issue of medication is important because it is so common as a treatment within mental health. Guidance from the National Institute of Clinical Excellence (NICE) states that the combination of medication and CBT is effective (NICE, 2009). Although this manual is concerned with CBT, it will be helpful to seek advice and guidance from your supervisor or manager about the effects of medication. Although medication can be an important element of treatment it is worthwhile striking a note of caution. Antidepressants do not provide a 'cure' for depression, they simply suppress the symptoms of the condition. A client may continue to take them after they have recovered in order to prevent depression from recurring. They do not, however, treat the psychological aspects of depression such as hopelessness, low self-esteem and lack of pleasure that we discussed earlier. Although the different methods of treatment, whether it is medication or psychotherapy, are important, the relationship that the worker has with a client is seen as the foundation in any mental health recovery (Gilbert & Leahy, 2007). This relationship will be looked at in more detail in Chapter 6. In the meantime it will help to begin to look at how we talk about depression with clients.

Talking about depression with clients

While the theory of depression is important, it is vital that we think about how this can be seen in practice. The background of depression is best explained by the client, who is the real expert of their own condition. It can be helpful when working with a client who has depression to gain a sense of what they think may have led them to experiencing the illness. See the dialogue below for an example.

Worker: *'Can you tell me what you think has led to you becoming depressed?'*

Client: *'I don't know.'*

Worker: *'Did it come on suddenly or was it gradual?'*

Client: *'I have been feeling like this for a few months now.'*

Worker: *'Ok. Can you remember if there was anything happening in your life at the time that may have impacted on you?'*

The client may have some idea what was occurring prior to their current situation but sometimes clients find it difficult to distinguish what may have led to it. It can sometimes help to prompt them.

Worker: *'Sometimes people with depression may find that there was something happening in their life around the time their symptoms started. We sometimes call these critical life events and examples may be things like a change in job, being made redundant, a relationship breakup or death of a loved one or friend. Has anything like this happened to you?'*

It is important when trying to explain a condition like depression to clients that you emphasise that the condition is an illness and not 'their fault'. This takes away some degree of shame from the individual. A client is more likely to work on their depression if they feel less ashamed.

Helplessness and powerlessness are aspects of depression. A way to help with this is to sit with the client and ask them about their symptoms of depression. Look at the example in the dialogue below.

Worker: *'Can you tell me how depression affects you, what are your particular signs and symptoms that you experience?'*

Client: *'I just feel like I have no energy, I don't look forward to anything and feel low all the time.'*

Worker: [you could try and prompt the client] *'How does it affect your sleep and your appetite?'*

Client: *'Oh I just want to sleep all the time and have no appetite anymore.'*

Once you feel that you have a sense of what the signs and symptoms are, you could then give them a copy of the symptoms of depression from Handout 2.1.

Worker: *'I would like to give you this sheet, which is what doctors use to diagnose someone with depression. What do you think of it?'*

Client: *'It describes some of my symptoms, yes.'*

Worker: *'Ok. Can you see that much of what you are experiencing is the symptoms of an illness and this is not your fault?'*

Client: *'Yes I can see that, although I still blame myself for not getting better.'*

The belief that it is the client's fault relates to some of the thoughts that people with depression have. Because of this it might be helpful to emphasise that they are symptoms of the illness and not personality defects.

In summary, depression affects every aspect of a person's life. Although this manual is about using CBT in working with depression, it is important to recognise that treatment is very often a team approach. The teams you work in will have many different types of staff, ranging from community psychiatric nurses to social workers. Their role can help in the range of social, environmental and financial factors which play a part in people's depression. The content of this chapter will hopefully prepare the ground for working with a client who is depressed. In the next chapter we will look at how this model of depression can be applied to the client in order for them to make sense of their story.

Exercise 2.1: Talking about depression for the first time

Think about the following questions (see Handout 2.1), record them in your journal and discuss with your supervisor or manager.

Talking about depression for the first time:

- How would you tell the difference between feeling low in mood and suffering from depression?
- How is being sad different from depression?
- How would you explain depression to a client?
- Can you identify any vulnerability factors for depression in your clients?
- If you work with someone who is depressed can you identify any other problems they may have?

Reflection

In your journal think about some of the following questions, and write down a few answers.

- *Have you or anyone you know suffered from depression? How did you know?*
- *What protects people from depression?*
- *Can you identify any vulnerability factors for yourself for depression?*

Conclusion

One of the problems with talking about depression as an illness is that it assumes that the person is in the grip of something which is outside of his or her control. This is not the case because changes in thinking and in particular activity can help a person to recover. These approaches are discussed in the next two chapters.

References

American Psychiatric Association (2013) *Diagnostic and Statistical Manual of Mental Disorders* (5th edition). Washington: American Psychiatric Association.

Beck AT, Rush AJ, Shaw BF & Emery G (1979) *Cognitive Therapy of Depression.* New York: Guilford Press.

Gilbert P & Leahy R (2007) *The Therapeutic Relationship In The Cognitive Behavioural Psychotherapies.* London: Routledge.

Judd LL (1997) The clinical course of unipolar major depressive disorders. *Archives of General Psychiatry* **54** 28–34.

Kendler KS, Karkowski LM & Prescott CA (1999) Causal relationship between stressful life events and the onset of major depression. *American Journal of Psychiatry* **156** 837–841.

Kupfer DJ (1991) Long-term treatment of depression. *Journal of Clinical Psychiatry* **52** (suppl. 5) 28–34.

NICE (2009) *Depression in Adults: Recognition and management.* Available at: https://www.nice.org.uk/guidance/CG90 (accessed December 2016).

World Bank (1993) *World Development Report: Investing in health research development.* Geneva, Switzerland: World Bank.

Handout 2.1

Exercise 2.1: Talking about depression for the first time

Think about the following questions and record them in your journal. Discuss them with your supervisor or manager.

- How would you tell the difference between feeling low in mood and suffering from depression?

- How is being sad different from depression?

- How would you explain depression to a client?

- Can you identify any vulnerability factors for depression in your clients?

- If you work with someone who is depressed can you identify any other problems they may have?

Symptoms of depression

1. **Depressed mood** – this means depressed for most of the day, nearly every day, as indicated by subjective report (i.e. what the individual client says) or observation by other people – family, friends or other professionals.

2. **Markedly diminished interest or pleasure** – the client experiences a loss of interest and pleasure in almost all activities most of the day, nearly every day.

3. **Physical symptoms** – this could be significant weight loss when not dieting, or weight gain. It might also include a decrease or increase in appetite nearly every day.

4. **Sleep** – the client may experience insomnia or excess sleep most days.

5. **Psychomotor agitation or retardation** – this term describes subjective feelings of restlessness or being slowed down. This may also be observed by others – family, friends or other professionals.

6. **Fatigue or loss of energy** – the client experiences these physical symptoms nearly every day.

7. **Thoughts about being worthless and feelings of excessive or inappropriate guilt** – the client with clinical depression can experience these thoughts and feelings nearly every day.

8. **Concentration** – the client's ability to think or concentrate is affected. They may feel unable to make a decision (again, this can be either subjective or observed by others).

9. **Recurrent thoughts of death** – this may include frequent ideas about suicide. This does not necessarily mean that they have a plan or intention to commit suicide.

Chapter 3: Formulation – the links between thoughts, feelings, physical sensations and behaviours in depression

Learning outcomes

By the end of this chapter you will be able to:

- help the individual client to understand their depression.

QCF units

Health and Social Care Diploma Level 3

- Unit SHC 31: Promote communication in health, social care or children's and young people's settings. Learning outcomes 1, 2, 3 and 4.

In the last chapter we discussed what can make people vulnerable to depression. We explored the cognitive model of depression (Beck *et al*, 1979) and how core beliefs and rules for living can be important. If you are working alongside a CBT therapist then one of the things they will have completed shortly after assessment will be the client's own individual formulation. The formulation is a working hypothesis of the client's own problems and how these may have developed, and can be a way of linking together the past and the present. It is likely that the cognitive model would have been used as a framework for this information. It may be helpful to speak with your supervisor about how they developed this formulation.

You could also work with your client in trying to develop a basic formulation. The object here is to get a shared understanding so that you as the worker, and the client, reach a consensus about what the problem is and how to tackle it.

Exercise 3.1: Formulation

Look at the following and work with the client on constructing their story.

The client's core beliefs will contain their view of how they see themselves, the world and their future. Remember that these beliefs are ingrained and will have developed at a very young age. You can explore with the client how they may have developed these beliefs by starting to talk about their early life experiences. It is important to note that this can be a very difficult area for clients to discuss depending on their background, and caution should be used.

The rules that clients develop to protect themselves from their core beliefs may provide a short-term solution as long as their circumstances support these beliefs. Remember these beliefs are inflexible, flexible beliefs can bend and adapt in relation to life circumstances. If beliefs are inflexible they can be easily broken by a variety of life situations. In the previous chapter we looked at core beliefs and rules and assumptions. In the example we used, a rule such as 'always keep working' was helpful for the client with a core belief of 'being a failure'. This rule is inflexible because it applies in all situations. It is a problem because in reality it can be easily broken, particularly when something arises which is outside of the client's control, such as redundancy. As you construct the client's story, enable them to make these connections if possible. Aim at using the client's own language and pick out words or phrases which appear to 'leap out'. Don't worry about whether the words seem over the top. Some examples might include 'in the pit', 'under a black cloud', 'caught between a rock and a hard place'.

There will be expressions which are particular to the client. When you have enough expressions, begin to try to develop them into a story. For example 'When I was a kid my family was…'.

Work with the client while writing down as much detail as you can. Use Handout 3.1 as a guide.

The bullet points in Handout 3.1 broadly outline the key areas to look at. When you have recorded some of this with the client take two steps back and think about the effect that all these experiences have had on the way that they think about themselves. Some clients may find it hard to recall their early life in detail, which is understandable. When we are young we are dependent and vulnerable, and anxious if we or our parents are threatened. If the relationship between the client's parents was threatening, i.e. they were physically violent, ask them how they coped, how they managed to keep safe. In this example the client may have coped by physically hiding away. Alternatively, the parents may not have been violent, but were just critical of the client which then affected their self-esteem. The threats here are less obvious and may be dealt with differently. The client may have coped by just keeping out of the way of their parents.

Think about the consequences of childhood experiences. If the client felt that their parents 'wrapped them in cotton wool', this could hamper their experience of the outside world. They could grow up feeling anxious and afraid of life and learn to not take risks. Ways of coping with early life problems may have made sense in the past but in the present may be part of the problem.

Think about the connections between core beliefs and ways of coping and see how far they are linked. For example:

'Because of feeling scared all of the time, I believed that I had to put on a brave face. This has led to me feeling as though I am acting when in the company of others, pretending to them that everything is ok.'

Make notes with the clients about these connections. The aim here will be to link together how the early life experience of the client led to them thinking about themselves, how they felt emotionally, how they tried to cope and finally how their ways of coping broke down. In CBT we sometimes use an approach which is like a flow diagram (see Figure 3.1).

Figure 3.1

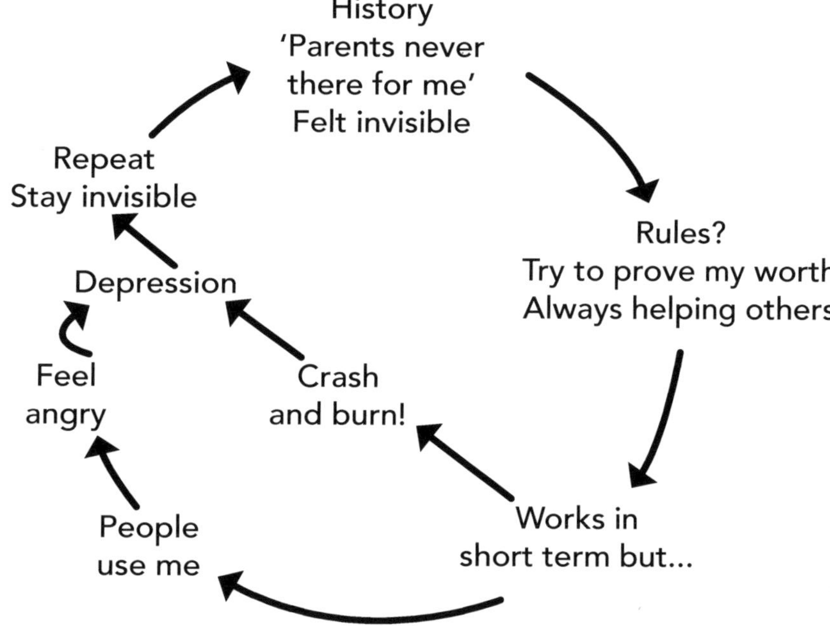

After doing this exercise, talk through the results with other professionals who may be involved in the care of the client. This could either be informally or through forums such as Care Programme Approach reviews. See how far the results of your assessment reflect the views and opinions of other professionals' assessments.

Assessments such as this are important in that they form the link between the roots of the client's problem in their early life experience, the beliefs they formed about themselves, how they coped, and how far this coping has reinforced the original problem.

Reflection

Enabling the client to re-write their story or to draw out their diagrams can sometimes provide a 'light bulb' moment in working with depression. Reflect on what the experience was like for you and then make a record in your journal.

References

Beck AT, Rush JA, Shaw BF, & Emery G (1979) *Cognitive Therapy for Depression.* New York: Guildford Press

Handout 3.1: Building up a picture of the client

1. **Early experiences**
   - Who were their parent figures and what was the relationship like between them?
   - Did they have brothers and sisters, and what was their relationship with them like?
   - Who were the extended family and what was the relationship like with them?
2. **School**
   - What was school like?
   - Did the client experience any bullying/was the client the bully?
   - Did the client have many friends and were they able to bring them home – if not, were there any reasons for this?
   - If the client did well at school, were their achievements recognised and praised by their parents?
3. **Work**
   - Was the client able to do the kind of work that they had always wanted to do?
   - What were relationships at work like?
   - How many jobs has the client had?
4. **Relationships**
   - Is the client currently in a relationship?
   - What is their relationship history?
5. **Culture**
   - Are there any relevant cultural issues?
   - What is the ethnicity of the client?

Chapter 4: Making sense of depression – thinking

Learning outcomes

By the end of this chapter you will:

- be able to identify Beck's triad of negative thoughts about self, the world and the future.
- be able to notice how depressed clients maintain depression by virtue of a process of distorted perception and memory recall.
- be familiar with the 10 Errors of Thinking. You will be able to use thought monitoring records to help clients capture negative thoughts and challenge them in order to arrive at more helpful, rational thoughts which improve mood.

QCF units

Health and Social Care Diploma Level 3

- Unit SHC 31: Promote communication in health, social care or children's and young people's settings. Learning outcomes 1, 2, 3 and 4.

While this manual looks at treatments that can be used with clients with depression in general, the main focus will be on clients who are suffering from chronic and severe depression.

Defining the severity of depression

In Chapter 2 we looked at the DSM-5 which described the symptoms of severe depression (American Psychiatric Association, 2013). In the DSM, phrases such as acute, chronic and severe are used to describe depression. These descriptions refer to a range of symptoms but also reflect how severe and persistent they might be. In CBT it is vital that our interventions are appropriate to the level of severity of the disorder and that we have a means of measuring progress. Because of this we need to be able to link the features of depression to a measure which is reliable and valid. The worker may come across a number of measures used in depression, such as the Beck Depression Inventory (Beck *et al*, 1996).

Capturing this individualised severity is essential in the process of formulating a treatment plan. A first step will be to refer back to Beck's depression model (Beck *et al*, 1979) mentioned in Chapter 2 with reference to the four aspects which are affected in depression: thinking, emotions/mood, physiology and behaviour. To use this with a client we start by enabling the client to recount what they experience when they are depressed and try to categorise these experiences as physiological, cognitive, emotional or behavioural. We aim to cluster their symptoms under these headings, on a sheet of paper using the Four Aspects of Self Model described below. Using different colours to describe each group of symptoms can help to reinforce these links and enable the client to recognise the wide reaching impact of depression on every aspect of themselves.

Exercise 4.1

Think of an occasion when you have been struggling with a particular life problem. Try to recall what you remember most vividly in terms of the impact this experience had on you. In doing so, see if you can identify which aspects of yourself were adversely affected. Now use the Four Aspects Model shown in Handout 4.1 to categorise the experiences. What you now have is a snapshot of your experience at that time and this can be a useful metaphor for clients when looking at their experience of being depressed.

The Four Aspects of Self Model is based on the work of Greenberger and Padesky (1995). Such models help us to see the way each aspect of the self interacts with all other parts. Clearly in the case of depression this interaction is negative. By using this model clients can begin to notice the interaction between their thoughts and their mood. In exploring a situation a client can be encouraged to notice that lowering of mood is linked to particular types of negative thoughts or images. With questioning, clients can be further enabled to notice that a vicious circle (see Figure 4.1) can emerge whereby lowered mood increases the frequency of negative thoughts and/or images, which then lowers mood and again increases negative cognitions and so on.

Figure 4.1

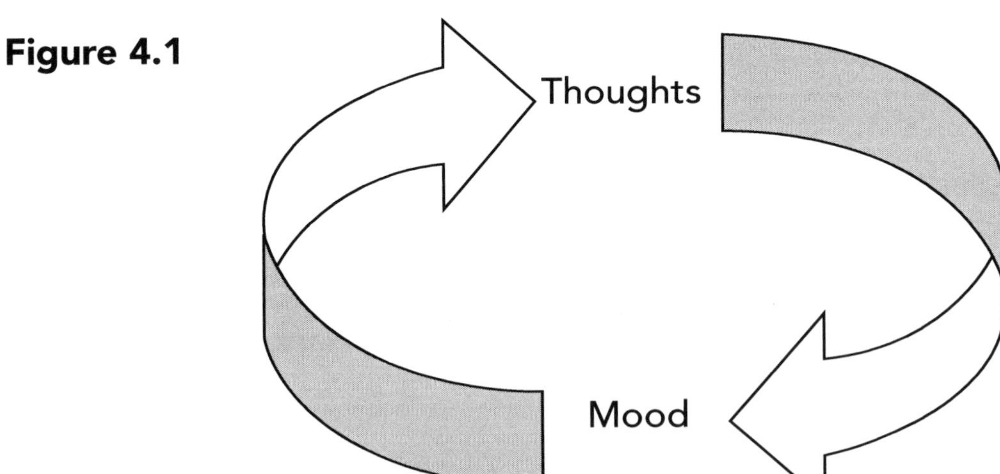

At this point we can ask clients which of the areas of their self they can have direct control over. Inevitably our thinking and our behaviour are the only things we can directly alter. Emotional and physiological changes are the consequences of our thinking and behaviour.

In Chapter 2 we explored the CBT model of depression as initially described by Beck *et al* (1979). Looking at this model we can see that the last stage in this model represents the symptoms of depression as they manifest in the four areas of the self (see p19). This is the client's experience of depression arising from the interplay between thought processes, which have been shaped by early life experiences and subsequent critical life events. The idea of the vicious circle is an important idea in working with CBT and depression. How it applies specifically to the client will be explored in Chapter 5.

In summary, we should educate clients to recognise that when depressed they can get caught in a self-maintaining vicious circle. CBT can help clients to get some perspective and help clients to detect negative automatic thoughts (NATS). They are automatic because they seem to 'pop' into our heads without choice, and they are negative because they are almost invariably bad in terms of what they do to our mood. The 10 Errors of Thinking are:

1. **Overgeneralisation.** Here we reach a conclusion based on one event or piece of evidence. Something bad occurs once and we expect it to happen repeatedly. Look out for the words 'always' and 'never' as signs. For example:

   'I forgot to finish the job on time. I never do things right.'

2. **Filtering (selective abstraction).** The focus is on the negatives and we ignore the positives or any information which might contradict our negative view of life.

   'The manager liked my work but pointed out a number of errors. He must think I am rubbish.'

3. **All or nothing/black and white thinking.** This is thinking in extremes – good/bad/right/wrong. There is no middle ground.

   'I made so many mistakes. If I can't do it perfectly I might as well not bother. I won't be able to get all of this done, so I may as well not start it. This job is so bad...there's nothing good about it at all.'

4. **Personalising.** Here we take on responsibility for something that's not our fault. We think that what people say or do is a kind of reaction to ourselves or is linked in some way to us.

   'John's in a terrible mood. It must have been something I did.'

   'It's obvious he doesn't like me, otherwise he would've said hello.'

5. **Catastrophising.** This is when we overestimate the risk of something bad happening. The key word here is 'overestimate'. The risk is usually not that bad.

   'I'm going to make a fool of myself and people will laugh at me.'

   'What if I haven't turned the iron off; the house will burn down.'

   'If I don't perform well, I'll get the sack.'

6. **Emotional reasoning.** Mistaking our feelings for facts. Negative things you feel about yourself are regarded as true because they feel true.

   'I feel guilty, I must have done something wrong.'

   'I feel anxious, something bad is going to happen.'

7. **Mind reading.** This is when we make negative assumptions about other people's thoughts, feelings and behaviours regarding us despite the lack of factual evidence.

   'If I see someone looking at me it means they think I'm ugly.'

   'I could tell he thought I was stupid when we first met.'

8. **Fortune telling.** Here we anticipate an outcome and assume that our prediction will come true. These negative expectations can work as self-fulfilling prophecies, as predicting what we would do on the basis of past behaviour may prevent the possibility of change.

   'There's no point going to the party as no-one will speak to me.'

   'I could never pass a driving test so why bother taking lessons?'

   'I've been asked out on a date but I can't go because I will make a fool of myself.'

9. **'Should' statements.** We end up using 'should', 'ought', or 'must' statements which then lead us to make unrealistic expectations of ourselves and other people. We end up living by rigid rules and not being flexible.

   'I shouldn't get angry.'

   'People should be nice to me all the time.'

10. **Magnification/minimisation.** Here we tend to exaggerate the importance of any negative experience while reducing the significance of positive information.

    'He noticed I spilled something on my shirt. I know he said he will go out with me again, but I bet he doesn't call.'

    'Supporting my friend when her mother died still doesn't make up for that time I got angry at her last year.'

These 'thinking errors' are one of the mechanisms which cause clients to notice and recall evidence/material which matches their depressed mood. They can appear to ignore or filter out and forget evidence which does not fit with their depressed state. It might be seen in the way that clients think about good and bad experiences. Bad experiences are seen as reflections of personal inadequacy or failure. The self-blame that follows thoughts of failure is remarkably consistent across situations and times.

For example, a 50-year-old client struggling to pay bills because of being out of work due to an unpredictable downturn in the economy perceives this as, 'Well I should have picked a better career when I left school – I wouldn't be in this mess then, would I?'

Should positive experiences be pointed out or indeed noticed, they will be dismissed as chance occurrences; a fluke specific to that time and place and certainly nothing to do with anything good or useful they may have done or could repeat.

The model of depression

Beck *et al* (1979) noted that his depressed clients often expressed negative thoughts in three domains or areas. He termed this the 'negative cognitive triad' as it reflected negative thoughts about the self, future and the world. These areas have been modified by subsequent authors. Moore and Garland (2003), in their work on chronic depression, refer to depression as a triangle of 'helplessness, hopelessness and low self-worth'. As a worker it can be helpful to look out for statements by clients which might reflect these three viewpoints.

We now need to consider a client's thinking style when depressed. In Chapter 2 we mentioned how the depression model explores early life experiences. These experiences give rise to what we call 'core beliefs'. These are fundamental beliefs that a person with depression has about themselves. They are expressed with usually just one word:

'I'm a failure.'

'I'm useless.'

'I'm defective.'

For clients with depression, intermediate beliefs – assumptions and life rules – are a way of managing these beliefs. They are often expressed as either 'if…then' statements:

'If I am in work, then I am not a failure.'

Or they are expressed as 'must' or 'should' statements:

'I must be useful/should be useful all of the time.'

Rules, assumptions and intermediate beliefs are, in the client's mind, inflexible. If they are broken by something which might be outside of the client's control, such as redundancy or bereavement (the 'critical incident' mentioned in the depression model), then there is no protection from the core beliefs. Negative automatic thinking is 'activated' and the depression cycle begins. In CBT it is recognised that core beliefs are difficult to identify but can be inferred from the nature of the intermediate beliefs. Some of the 'question asking' techniques outlined in Chapter 1 can be helpful here. The change that we can bring about is linked to the idea of the 'content and process' of depressed thinking.

Content

As stated earlier, depressed thinking tends to consist of negative thoughts regarding the self, the world (and people in it) and the future. Typically, a client will express views about being weak or inadequate, how other people are normal or better than them and that they do not have a future or, if they do, it is a bleak one.

Process

These negative thoughts are produced and maintained by distortions in the perception and memory of the client. In practice this will be the negative automatic thinking demonstrated above.

Therapy

At the start it is important to teach clients how to identify their own negative automatic thoughts. In doing this it is important to remember that not all negative automatic thoughts are wrong. For example, someone who has been made redundant from work and believes their income will decrease resulting in an inability to maintain payments on their mortgage or new car, would not be 'catastrophising'. Thoughts such as these are factual and would need a problem-solving approach. However if the client voices a belief that they have lost their job and will 'never' be able to work again, then this invites closer questioning as it may be a distortion. Once you have an idea of the type of thoughts that the client may be using, it becomes helpful to put the thought 'on trial'. By this we mean asking the client to come up with evidence which either supports or disproves the belief.

As we said earlier, this is often difficult as when positive experiences do occur they are often dismissed as 'flukes'. Because of this it will be important to emphasise that this is not the client being stupid or awkward; it is a symptom of depression that arises automatically with the condition. A useful tool for your client in working with NATS is a thought monitoring and challenging record.

Thought monitoring record

Our primary instrument for helping clients with unhelpful cognitions is a form known as a thought monitoring record (see Handout 4.2). Different authors and practitioners have modified these to suit either particular clients or to satisfy their own preferences, but they all generally follow a similar format (Beck *et al*, 1979).

Exercise 4.2

Use a copy of Handout 4.2 on yourself. Rate the percentage of intensity of the emotion/mood/feeling and the percentage of belief that you may have in your thinking. The closer you get to 100% belief the more certain you are in the thought. Keep a record of this in your journal.

Reflection

A frequent difficulty in completing such forms is not being able to name emotions. The confusion between emotions and thoughts will be detailed in the next section. In the meantime it may help to look at the handout at the end of this section (Handout 4.4) which references the emotions. In your journal, write about how your experience of

Exercise 4.2 was. Was it helpful or unhelpful? Easy or difficult? Now consider how this would be experienced by the clients you are working with who have depression. Given the problems that depression brings, what difficulties could you foresee?

Exercise 4.3

It is possible in reflecting on Exercise 4.2 that you may be concerned that your clients might have difficulty in working with the format. In view of this, we can start by using an abridged version of the form (see Handout 4.3), which only uses the first three columns of the full form. When using this form, ask the client to bring to mind a recent situation or event which led to a noticeable drop in mood. To help identify the negative automatic thought which might lie behind the drop in mood ask the client to give details about the event.

- Where did it happen?
- When did it happen?
- Who else was involved?
- What exactly occurred?

The answers to these questions will form the content of the first column of the thought record.

Next we move to the emotions/mood column. You may find that the client confuses thoughts and emotions.

For example the expression:

'I felt stupid.'

Stupid is not an emotion but is a thought and you could helpfully rephrase the statement more accurately as:

'I believe I am stupid' or 'I am stupid.'

It will be helpful to examine the handout on emotions (see Handout 4.4), which gives a basic description of five key emotions and the idea of different phrases referring to different levels of intensity of emotion. This will help the client to complete the percentage rating of the intensity of the feeling.

Finally we come to the column for recording thoughts, which also includes mental images or memories. At this point the worker is looking for comments which reflect negative views about the self, the type of world they see around them and their future. Again the client is asked to estimate their intensity of belief in the thought and express it as a percentage. It is important to be systematic when helping the client to fill this in to ensure that each identified emotion is clearly linked to a particular thought. This will help to separate out the specific depressive thoughts from ones linked to anxiety, guilt and shame.

Reflection

Having tried this format of a thought record with one of your clients, consider how you might extend your skills and introduce them to the seven column sheet in Handout 4.2. Look at the completed seven column example for Eric (Handout 4.5) before working with the blank sheet with yourself, and then the client (Handout 4.6).

In the example of Eric we can see that, despite successfully challenging his negative thoughts, he is still sad. Thought records will not provide an overnight cure for depression but what is important to highlight is the reduction in the percentage intensity of the sadness; 40% compared to 70% in this case.

Intermediate beliefs and behavioural experiments

Finally we come to working with intermediate beliefs; the assumptions and rules that can play such an important role in the avoidance response in depression. Thought challenging has a vital role in this aspect of treating depression but can be massively enhanced by the application of 'behavioural experiments' (Bennett-Levy *et al*, 2004).

A difficulty that we may run up against with a client such as Eric will be a tendency to use terms such as 'yes, but...'. Each time a challenge to his way of thinking has been made, he may respond with any number of reasons why it may not work. How might we challenge his negative predictions about attending the wedding? What can help here is looking at 'behavioural experiments'. This is a way of setting up a situation which tests the negative thought in question.

If we look at Eric's thought record, his key thoughts about the wedding revolve around predictions regarding what he believes people will think about him or how they may treat him. Embedded in this prediction is an assumption that, as he is unemployed, he is not as worthy as other people and even his close friends will reject him. Eric needs to test this theory out because at the moment he really believes it to such an extent he will not go to the wedding. There are four simple steps to a behavioural experiment:

1. Planning. What activity will enable Eric to check out his belief?
2. Predict. What is Eric's prediction about what will happen in the experiment? Get him to give the prediction a percentage probability rating.
3. Undertake the experiment.
4. Compare the actual outcome with the original prediction.

The intermediate belief that Eric is going to check out is the assumption that others will reject him because he is unemployed. In discussion with his worker they agree that a valid test would be for Eric to arrange to meet socially with Dave and a few mutual friends.

Eric predicts that if they agree to meet they will not engage with him much or just ignore him. Eric gives this a probability rating of 80%. In addition, the therapist asked

Eric to predict how much he would enjoy the event. Eric gave a prediction rating of 5%. Fortunately the social event happened and Eric met with his worker to discuss the results of the experiment.

Worker: *So Eric, you met up with your friends, how did it go?'*

Eric: *'Well I have to admit I feel an utter fool about what I said would happen. I was nervous at first but everyone was genuinely pleased to see me and I was totally included in the conversation. And funnily enough, some of the chaps still working at my old place said they envied me being made redundant because it's awful working there now.'*

Worker: *'How accurate would you say your prediction of being ignored was?'*

Eric: (laughing) *'Totally inaccurate, I was not ignored at all and really enjoyed myself. In fact we've arranged to try and meet up once a month after Dave's got the wedding out of the way.'*

Worker: *'Can you give me a rating of how enjoyable it was?'*

Eric: *'Oh, off the scale, 110%; I haven't enjoyed myself so much in ages.'*

Worker: *'What thoughts do you have about attending the wedding?'*

Eric: *'Now I've checked it out I'll be fine. Obviously there will be people there I don't know so I might be a bit guarded in my conversation but I know my mates still value me so that's okay.'*

Exercise 4.4

Using the dialogue above, think about the type of behavioural experiment you might use with a client. Set up a situation with a client where you can test a negative automatic thought. Discuss the results in supervision with your manager or supervisor.

Reflection

With the above exercise remember that whatever the outcome of the behavioural experiment, the results will be important. If it does not work, the reasons for any failure will help in understanding the barriers to change. A final comment regarding any interaction with clients is the need to practise the skill of open questioning in supervision. This skill was dicussed in Chapter 1. However, it needs to be emphasised how much this skill is threaded throughout the whole of this manual. When working with clients it is more helpful to ask questions with a sense of gentle curiosity rather than in the style of an interrogator.

References

American Psychiatric Association (2013) *Diagnostic and Statistical Manual of Mental Disorders* (5th edition). Washington: American Psychiatric Association.

Beck AT, Rush AJ, Shaw BF & Emery G (1979) *Cognitive Therapy of Depression.* New York: Guilford Press.

Beck AT, Steer RA, Ball R & Ranieri W (1996) Comparison of Beck Depression Inventories -IA and II in psychiatric outpatients. *Journal of Personality Assessment* **67** (3) 588–597.

Bennett-Levy, Butler G, Fennel M, Hackmann M, Mueller M & Westbrook D (Eds) (2004) *Oxford Guide to Behavioural Experiments in Cognitive Therapy*. Oxford: Oxford University Press.

Greenberger D & Padesky CA (1995) *Mind over Mood: Change how you feel by changing the way you think*. New York: Guilford Press.

Moore R & Garland A (2003) *Cognitive Therapy for Chronic and Persistent Depression*. Chichester: Wiley.

Handout 4.1

Exercise 4.1: Four Aspects of Self Model

Thoughts	Emotions	Physiology	Behaviour

Handout 4.2

Exercise 4.2: Thought monitoring record

Event	Emotion/ mood/feeling	Negative Automatic Thought (NAT) (Image/ Memory)	Evidence that supports the NAT	Evidence that contradicts the NAT	What's a more balanced alternative view to take?	Any change in mood?
	% intensity	% belief				

Handout 4.3

Exercise 4.3: Abridged thought monitoring record

Event	Mood/emotion	Thought
	% Intensity	% of Belief

Handout 4.4

Exercise 4.4: Brief summary of emotions

Anger

This emotion arises when we encounter an injustice against ourselves or those we care about. A moral rule is seen as being broken and we are stimulated to remedy the unfairness. This is an activating emotion which invites us to approach the problem and sort it out.

Frustrated Annoyed Angry Furious Raging

|---|

0% 100%

Fear

This emotion arises when we are feeling threatened and do not have the resources to protect ourselves or others we care about. It too is an activating emotion but it drives us to run away, escape or avoid similar situations in the future.

Apprehensive Nervous Frightened Panicky Terrified

|---|

0% 100%

Disgust

This emotion arises when we are revolted or repelled by something. It is an activating emotion which drives us to distance ourselves from the object of revulsion either by moving away from it or by discarding it. Surprisingly it lacks a wide range of words to describe the intensity of the emotion. Closely associated with the feeling of hatred.

Distaste Revulsion Abject disgust

|---|

0% 100%

Sadness

This emotion usually arises in the context of perceived or actual loss. It may be loss of material objects, status or relationships. It is a deactivating emotion which invites us to become paralysed with inertia and hunker down. It is the emotion most commonly experienced in depression.

Fed up Down Quite low Sad Despondent Utter despair

|---|

0% 100%

Handout 4.4
Exercise 4.4: Brief summary of emotions (continued)

Guilt

This is an emotion which arises when we believe we have caused harm to others, either by doing something or failing to do something. When experienced it motivates us to make reparations to whoever we have harmed. Unfortunately in depression it can be activated by errors of thinking so is regarded as inappropriate guilt.

|--|

0% 100%

Shame

Shame is a fear-based emotion and arises when we believe we are seen as inferior, flawed or an object of disgust by other people. It motivates us to hide away from those we believe will see us in this way due to fear of rejection, ridicule or worse.

|--|

0% 100%

Handout 4.5

Event	Emotion % belief	Negative Automatic Thought (NAT) (Image/memory) % belief	Evidence to support the thought (NAT)	Evidence that contradicts the thought (NAT) Any thinking errors?	What's a more balanced alternative view to take? % belief	Any change in mood? % intensity
Wedding invitation	Sadness. 70% belief	This is my life from now on. Trapped, never able to take part in a normal social life again. I'm on the scrap heap and people in a job like Dave won't want someone they see as a benefit scrounger mixing with them. Everyone will ignore me if I go. 100% belief.	It's harder to get a job at my age. You read in the papers about politicians and everyone criticising the unemployed. Dave's probably no different deep down. I must be a scrounger. I can't pull myself together to apply for a job.	In some jobs that might be true but my years of experience make me an asset to the right company. Only certain papers make cheap shots at the unemployed. Others emphasise the effects of the economy. I've known Dave for years and I know he really values me as a friend. I'm claiming benefits I'm entitled to and which I've paid towards in tax. I can't help being depressed and I am working on it in therapy. When I'm able I will start looking for work. I'm catastrophising, fortune telling and mind reading.	Dave knows I'm out of work and struggling with depression. He would never try to shame me and a few more of our friends who he will invite are unemployed at the moment as well. Him and Jane have been together a couple of years so they don't really need big presents. I will go to the wedding!!	Excited 60% Sad 40%

Handout 4.6

Event	Emotion % belief	Negative Automatic Thought (NAT) (Image/ memory) % belief	Evidence to support the thought (NAT)	Evidence that contradicts the thought (NAT) Any thinking errors?	What's a more balanced alternative view to take? % belief	Any change in mood? % intensity

Chapter 5: Making sense of depression – activity

Learning outcomes

By the end of this chapter you will be able to:

- see the links between thoughts, emotions, physiology and behaviour in depression.
- use activity scheduling to develop behavioural plans to improve mood and reverse the vicious circle of negative thoughts that lower mood.
- use behavioural activation as a means to overcome avoidance.

QCF units

Health and Social Care Diploma Level 3

- Unit SHC 31: Promote communication in health, social care or children's and young people's settings. Learning outcomes 1, 2, 3 and 4.

A cognitive approach which involves clients learning to challenge unhelpful and inaccurate thoughts can be a highly effective therapeutic approach. However, it will often be the case that severely depressed clients struggle to use such techniques. It could present the risk of triggering negative thoughts about failure if unsuccessful. In view of this, it can be a more helpful first step to take a more behavioural route to improving the client's mood. Small increases in a client's behaviour levels can lead to improvements in mood. Sharing this observation with clients will often be met with comments like:

'I know that might help if I could do that, but I've got no energy or motivation to do it.'

Such comments are more likely to be reflecting the very real physical changes that arise in people when depressed. Their fatigue is real and reflects how people are less efficient when they are stressed. Furthermore, as perhaps noted in the Four Aspects Model presented earlier, food intake and sleep quality can suffer badly when one is depressed, which contributes to fatigue and lethargy.

With this in mind we need to recognise that while improvements in a client's overall activity levels may be helpful, achieving this increase can be a challenge. As such, we need to think carefully about how we use this method to greatest effect.

Behavioural activation

Behavioural activation is an approach which tries to get clients to focus on activities which are pleasurable and/or give a sense of accomplishment or achievement (Martell *et al*, 2010).

The initial phase involves introducing the client to an activity log or diary sheet which asks clients to note every day for a week what they do every hour, and to rate how depressed they feel on a scale of 0-10 with 0 being the least depressed and 10 being the most depressed. This task looks simple, but remember the client is depressed and likely to struggle with even the simplest of tasks at present.

Exercise 5.1

As with previous exercises it can help to use the techniques on yourself. Use a blank diary/log sheet (see Handout 5.1) and complete it over the next week. You can rate feelings of depression using the 0-10 score above. You may also choose an alternative mood such as anxiety or any other moods.

Reflection

Having completed this record, think about the following questions and write down your responses in your journal.

- Were there any patterns in the activity – were the mornings, afternoons or evenings better?
- Did some environments help more than others?
- Was it helpful being with people/being alone?

Look at your answers and think about how far these might reflect the patterns with clients. Make notes in your journal and discuss with your manager or supervisor.

Exercise 5.2

Go through the diary sheet then demonstrate its use by helping the client to fill it in for that day up to meeting with yourself (see Handout 5.1). Ask questions about how they 'felt' when doing these activities. This begins the process of enabling clients to link activities to mood. Once the client is clear about how to fill in the diary sheet, they are asked to complete one for the following week (see Handout 5.2). Ask the client to state what their mood was on completing the activity and to give it a rating, for example 0/10: not depressed and 10/10: very depressed. Ask them to bring it to the next session for discussion.

In reviewing a client's diary sheet it can help to begin with a general query as to whether there were variations in mood throughout the duration of the days. If this was the case, ask the client to consider that there may be patterns to the fluctuations in mood and to see if these fluctuations are linked to particular activities. See how far the client can recognise that some activities increase depressed mood and some activities lessen it.

Reflection

Reflect on how successful or unsuccessful the above activity was in your journal. If it was successful, consider extending the timetable into the evening i.e. from 5.00pm onwards. Now look at the following transcript between a client and worker when reviewing a diary sheet.

Worker: *'I see here you mention beginning to change the bed linen and recording your depressed mood as low at 8/10.'*

Client: *'It was just too much so I gave up. I felt a bit disappointed but generally my mood lifted a bit.'*

Worker: *'This seems to happen with a number of domestic activities like vacuuming and washing the dishes. It pushes your mood down when you start these tasks and when you give up it seems you feel better.'*

Client: *'Yeah it's pretty much the case that I feel better avoiding chores and it's been like that for a while now.'*

Think of the following question. Does the worker suggest to the client that as chores lower his mood it would be therapeutic to avoid such activities?

When treating depression, clinicians need to be aware that that there is a particularly unhelpful interaction between negative thoughts, avoidant behaviour and physiological inertia. This last concept refers to the notion that, when depressed, the mind and body seem to resist any effort to change from a state of inactivity to action. We can represent this in the Depression Pentagon model shown in Figure 5.1.

Figure 5.1

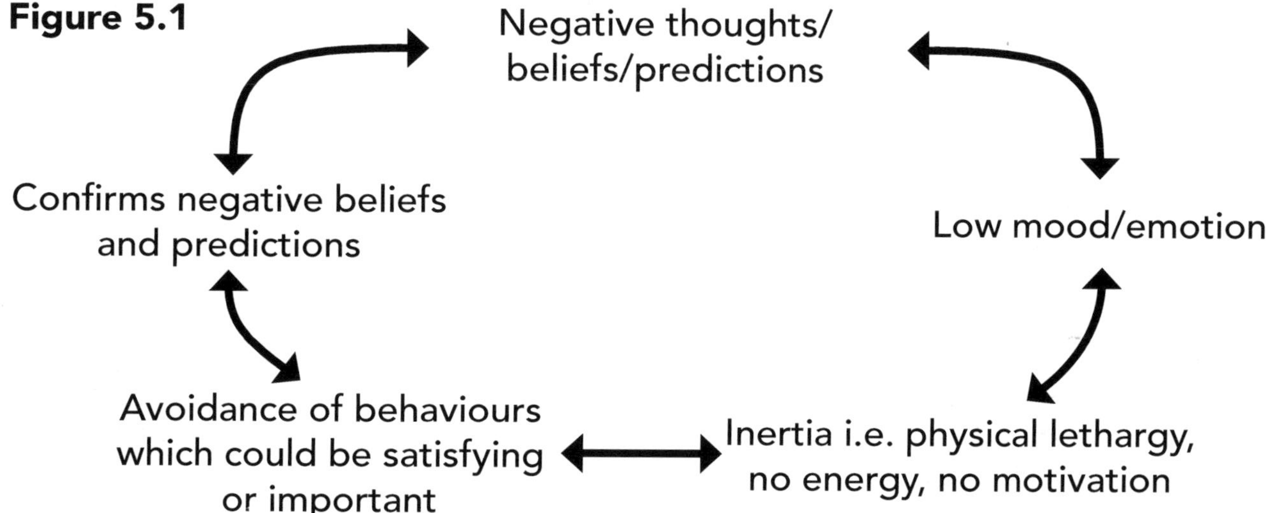

In view of this, the worker needs to ask the client about the possible negative consequences of avoidance.

Reflection

It is important to avoid making suggestions to the client, so try to focus on questions which can enable the client to reach their own answers. Look at using the techniques around open questions from Chapter 1. At first the client may see avoidance as something positive, in that at one level it can help to make them feel better. It can be useful to draw a distinction between what makes someone feel safe and what is helpful. Although freedom from anxiety may help, the longer term consequences for the client will be depression. A way of explaining in more detail how this works is the idea of reinforcement.

Reinforcement

At this point it may help to introduce the idea of reinforcement. Reinforcement is an idea from behavioural science which says that if an activity repeatedly provides a reward we are more likely to do it again and again. The activity therefore becomes reinforcing. People will continue to go to work because of the obvious reinforcement of receiving a wage. Reinforcement has two sides to it:

- Negative reinforcement. The reward is that a 'bad feeling is taken away'. Someone who is anxious about being with people will avoid crowds. The reinforcement will be that their anxiety levels will drop.
- Positive reinforcement. The reward is that a positive feeling is provided. The positive reinforcement of work is a wage. The positive reinforcement of sport is an increase in physical health.

This idea is important because on a fundamental level depression can be caused by a reduction in activities which provide positive reinforcement. Activity may therefore be a problem for a client with depression. It may help to inform the client that, as paradoxical as it might sound, the lethargy of depression is not the same as the lethargy we feel after hard physical work. The latter state requires rest whereas the lethargy of depression requires activity. As the client and worker continue examining the diary sheet, the worker will be looking for evidence that less depressed mood is linked to certain activities. These can be classed as those which are simply enjoyable and give a sense of pleasure, and those activities which, although not directly enjoyable, do give a sense of accomplishment or achievement (sometimes referred to as mastery). Look at the following dialogue:

Worker: *'Ok, let's carry on and look at some of these other activities and how you have rated their impact on your mood. Now this item I find really interesting. You noted that you were on the phone for over an hour arguing with your niece's insurance company trying to get a refund for her.*

You rated what I would class as a very stressful event as actually improving your mood resulting in a score of 2/10 for depressed mood. Can you say how this came about?'

Client: (laughs) *'Oh yeah, that was good. Well, I used to work for an insurance broker so I knew my niece had a good case. But obviously she lacked my knowledge so wouldn't be able to argue with the company. I was listening to her on the phone and could tell she was getting the brush off so got her permission to talk to them. They tried it with me but once I started quoting the law and regulations they soon put me onto someone more senior. They realised I was right and they gave my niece her refund.'*

Worker: *'Sounds like that felt good.'*

Client: *'Oh yes, excellent.'*

This as an example of a mastery activity – mastery in the sense that the client derived a great sense of achievement and success from using his knowledge and skills to help his niece. As this is such a good example of a mastery activity, you would be wise to use this to illustrate the concept to your clients.

Having grasped the idea of what a mastery activity involves, you could ask the client to rate how great a sense of accomplishment or satisfaction they derived from the activity. The client could use a 0 to 10 scale where 10 indicates an enormous sense of satisfaction and 0 no satisfaction at all. With this in mind, worker and client can go through the rest of the log sheet trying to identify other activities which may be regarded as mastery ones and to rate them out of 10.

The next step is to see whether there is a link between lower depressive mood scores and activities with high mastery scores. This again is a typical positive relationship and we would expect to see this in the client's log.

Having noted all the mastery activities you should look for times when other types of activity were engaged in but which also gave lower depressive mood scores. Let us continue to see how this might be explored:

Worker: *'I see here that there are four events you describe as 'watching telly' that gave a depressive mood rating of 3/10. Can you tell me a bit more about that?'*

Client: *'Well I'm a bit of a sci-fi addict and I love watching stuff like Star Trek or Dr Who. It's just escapism. A bit of a waste of time really but I do enjoy it.'*

Worker: *'So, not much mastery is required for this but it still helps your mood.'*

Client: *'Nope, no mastery but good fun.'*

Worker: *'That's good because in CBT we look for activities which give a sense of accomplishment, but also activities which are just simply enjoyable or pleasurable. I wonder if we can go through the log and see if there are other activities which are relatively enjoyable and see if they are related to better mood.'*

A review of the log will hopefully show a few activities that are pleasurable, give a sense of accomplishment or both, and will be generally linked to better mood scores. Activity diaries/logs provide a rich supply of material with which you can begin to undertake a behavioural assessment leading to a behavioural plan containing therapeutic goals.

Behavioural assessment

This involves using the diary sheet as a tool for getting a sense of what activities the client values and how this may be used to formulate therapeutic goals. In doing so, both client and worker get additional data regarding what activities are being avoided, what activities are being done too frequently and need decreasing and what activities might usefully be increased.

Activity planning

From this type of analysis of the log the client can be enabled to develop a plan which incorporates the above findings. In particular, establishing a weekly schedule of planned activities which have a positive impact on mood and begin to reduce inertia stemming from avoidance. It is vital when helping the client to plan their schedule that they are encouraged to engage in a variety of activities, which would involve:

- being social, engaging with others
- being by one's self
- different environments e.g. being at home or visiting somewhere else; this could be indoors or outside
- varying the time of day activities are carried out.

Furthermore, although some creativity and thinking outside the box can become useful, at first it is best to follow these principles:

- Keep it simple; too ambitious a plan will be unachievable and failure could derail the plan from the outset.
- If there are financial implications ensure the tasks are affordable. Remember the client may be on benefits or reduced income due to being off work with depression.
- Despite the client seeming to have large periods of time doing nothing, there may still be crucial activities being engaged in. Planned activities need to be easy to accommodate in the client's daily schedule.
- Do not suggest to or agree to the client engaging in activities which are patently outside of the client's ability.

Even with the above criteria in mind, it is easy to see a plan which, on the surface, seems to contain a selection of rewarding activities. See Figure 5.2 below for an example.

Figure 5.2

Thursday	
Time	**Activity**
8.00	Have breakfast
9.00	Wash up
10.00	Do some gardening
11.00	
12.00	Have lunch
1.00	Wash up
2.00	
3.00	Collect grandchild from school
4.00	Take grandchild out shopping to get something for tea
5.00	

This schedule would benefit from being more specific. This could be achieved if the worker asked the client to provide information regarding the who with, when and for how long, where, what exactly and to what extent. Now look at the following dialogue.

Worker: *'I see here, John, that you intend to do some gardening at 10.00. Would that be by yourself?'*

Client: *'Well, my wife enjoys gardening as well so we would both be in the garden.'*

Worker: *'I recall you saying that your relationship had suffered badly due to your being depressed so I wonder if gardening together might be a start to repairing this rift between you.'*

Client: *'I think so, it's been dreadful for both of us and I just feel good at the prospect of sharing an activity with Jane other than arguing.'*

Worker: *'Definitely something that's in tune with your values and a step towards that goal of getting your relationship back to how it used to be.'*

Client: *'I hope so.'*

Worker: *'Good. Now this phrase 'Gardening' is a bit general. I wonder if we could narrow it down to some specific tasks.'*

Client: *'Yes; the hedge needs trimming, the lawn needs cutting and the rockery needs weeding.'*

Worker: *'Hmm. That sounds like quite a lot of work; would you realistically expect to get all that done in one go?'*

Client: *'I could try, see how far I get.'*

Worker: *'That's certainly one approach to consider, but I wonder how you would feel if you didn't finish all the gardening you set out to do?'*

Client: *'Hmm, probably remind myself how useless I have become.'*

Worker: *'Ah! And what might that do to your mood?'*

Client: *'Not improve it for sure; no, it would make me feel a lot worse.'*

Worker: *'I suspect you are probably right, so can we see how we might make this a bit more manageable?'*

Client: *'Ok, I'm open to suggestions.'*

Worker: *'Right, now bearing in mind your mood and energy levels, how long do you think it would be reasonable to spend gardening?'*

Client: *'I could probably manage a couple of hours.'*

Worker: *'In view of how fatigued you are, two hours sounds a bit ambitious. How about starting with a half hour?'*

Client: *'Tch! Hardly worth getting my boots on for that length of time.'*

Worker: *'Ok what would be a reasonable compromise?'*

Client: *'At least an hour.'*

Worker: *'Fair enough, an hour. Now let's decide what specifically you will be doing.'*

Client: *'In an hour I reckon I can cut the lawn and rake up the loose cuttings.'*

Worker: *'Ok and now when do you plan to do it in terms of what day and starting time?'*

Client: *'Well the forecast is fine for tomorrow so I can do it then.'*

Worker: *'I know you struggle to get up early so what would be a reasonable start time?'*

Client: *'Oh, if I've got a reason to get up I can do. Erm, let's say 10.00, no 10.30, that should be ok.'*

Worker: *'Well this sounds like a reasonable plan. So, can I summarise it just to be sure we have covered everything. At 10.30 tomorrow you will join Jane in the garden and spend an hour cutting the lawn and raking up the loose cuttings. So we know what you will be doing, where you will be doing it, when and who you will be doing it with AND how long you will be doing it for.'*

The final planned activity is a collaborative activity between worker and client and is very specific. This same process would then be applied to perhaps two or three other activities related to items picked up from the original activity log.

Reflection

It may be the case that any planning that is done with a client may not be totally successful. This is to some extent inevitable, as depression is a complex condition. Make a note of this in your journal and discuss this with your supervisor or manager. Flexibility is important as a mental health worker in order to help clients 'move on' in treatment. Look at the next dialogue which reviews how the plan worked out for the client.

Client: *'Before you ask, I'm just going to confess that I blew it. I was a complete wash out.'*

Worker: *'You sound dejected. What happened?'*

Client: *'I got up fine, felt quite enthusiastic, went to the shed to get the lawn mower and saw it was a bit buried under some garden furniture. I went to move it and a chair got jammed and I just thought, "everything always goes against me, why bother?" and I burst into tears. I went back inside and spent a couple of hours staring at the wall and telling myself how utterly useless I am.'*

Worker: *'That sounds like a major knock-back, what about the other activities we identified?'*

Client: *'No good, just thought I've blown it, why bother? Spent all week going over all the things I've messed up and the people I've let down.'*

Before we can come up with a flexible approach we need to be clear about what has gone wrong. There are two tools we can consider here.

The first, TIAVOR (Trigger Interpretation AVOidance Response), describes a number of unhelpful behaviours we see often in depression. In the above example the client's trigger was the unexpected delay or extra effort needed to free the mower, which caused an eruption of negative automatic thinking that resulted in him abandoning the agreed task. The worker could ask the client to fill in a TIAVOR form (see Handout 5.3).

Exercise 5.3

When filling this out, the client could be asked if a short-term consequence of his avoidance would be his garden becoming increasingly wild. On recognising this the client will in all likelihood engage in an aggressive dialogue full of self-blaming comments. This response style is typical in people with depression.

Reflection

Consider the client's answers to Exercise 5.3 in the light of what you already know about the patterns of thinking within depression. It is likely that the client's mood will be pushed lower and his depression is either maintained or worsened. This may be the result of being self-critical because of a failure to do the gardening. Think about how the client may resolve this problem, and note down your thoughts before proceeding to Exercise 5.4.

Exercise 5.4

Getting the client 'back on course' can be helped by using the TIALTER form (Trigger, Interpretation, ALTErnative Response), where the alternative response is a helpful behaviour which has both positive short- and long-term consequences (see Handout 5.4).

By reviewing the trigger event, John could be asked to consider what would have been more helpful immediately after he walked away from the shed. Ideas such as having a cup of tea then returning to the task might have some merit! An appraisal of the benefits of this alternative to avoidance would be the elements of mastery and pleasure derived from the planned activity which we predicted would improve his mood in the short term. It would also contribute to his overcoming the inertia which would otherwise be reinforced by his avoidance, affecting long-term recovery from depression.

Reflection

The ultimate aim of activity monitoring and activity planning is to reduce unhelpful styles of thinking and acting, such as rumination and avoidance, and replace them with routines which are pleasurable, giving a sense of accomplishment. For many clients this behavioural approach will provide rich benefits in a relatively short time. However, for some people a behavioural approach is almost impossible to access due to the disabling power of their negative thoughts. How far have these ideas been useful in your work? Compare and contrast the approaches used here with the approaches used in the previous chapter. It will also help to revisit the section on goal setting from Chapter 1, which looked at activities that were positively reinforcing.

References

Martell CR, Dimidjian S & Herman-Dunn R (2010) *Behavioural Activation for Depression: A clinician's guide.* New York: Guilford Press.

Handout 5.1

Exercise 5.1: Day activity log

Day:	
Time	**Activity**
8.00	
9.00	
10.00	
11.00	
12.00	
1.00	
2.00	
3.00	
4.00	
5.00	

Handout 5.2

Exercise 5.2: Week activity log

	Monday	Tuesday	Wednesday	Thursday	Friday	Saturday	Sunday
8.00-9.00							
9.00-10.00							
10.00-11.00							
11.00-12.00							
12.00-1.00							
1.00-2.00							
2.00-3.00							
3.00-4.00							
4.00-5.00							

Handout 5.3

Exercise 5.3: TIAVOR form

Trigger event	Interpretation	Avoidance response	Short-term consequences of avoidance	Long-term consequences of avoidance

Handout 5.4

Exercise 5.4: TIALTER form

Trigger event	Interpretation	Avoidance response	Likely short-term consequences of alternative response	Likely long-term consequences of alternative response

Chapter 6: The therapeutic relationship

Learning outcomes

By the end of this chapter you will:

- be able to apply the tools of CBT to your own practice.
- have gained insight into the strengths and weaknesses of your practice.

QCF units

Health and Social Care Diploma Level 3

- Unit SHC 32 : Engage in personal development in health, social care or children's and young people's settings. Learning outcomes 1, 2, 3 ,4 and 5.

All of us have two sides to ourselves. This comes out when we refer to ourselves using the words 'I' or 'me'. We learn how to use 'me' as a reaction to our relationships with other people. Other people's attitudes about us become part of us. For example, if a lot of people appeared to treat me as if I am a failure from an early age, then I will eventually believe that I am one. People learn to see who they are by observing how others respond to them. You may have gained a sense of this while looking at the formulation from Chapter 3. However, when we speak of ourselves using the word 'I' we are more proactive. We are literally in the 'driving seat' of our lives.

'I drive my car.'

'I cook a meal.'

'I go to work.'

We also have a relationship with ourselves. Our self-to-self-relationship may mean that the 'I' gets angry with the 'me' because of its perceived failure.

If this belief is particularly intense we may look at our relationship with other people to see if it confirms what we think about ourselves. In the above example, we may be overly vigilant to signs that other people believe we are a failure because it will confirm what we think about ourselves.

We as the worker believe that we are helping the client. However, our help may then backfire and be perceived by the client as criticising, leaving them with a sense of powerlessness. As workers we need to have an awareness of how far these patterns may get reflected in our relationship with clients. How far are we secretly criticising clients? If the client believes that they have failed how far will they look to you as their worker for signs that they have failed? How far will their attempts to gain power be seen as resisting your help?

Understanding how we can play these roles in the relationship we have with ourselves and with clients is important (Wilde McCormick, 2008). We will be applying some of the CBT ideas to ourselves as workers. In order to understand this it will be useful to revisit errors of thinking from Chapter 4.

Exercise 6.1: Errors of thinking

As a starting point it may be useful to look at the errors of thinking from Chapter 4 (p33) and think about how far they might apply in your work with the client.
As workers we will also commit errors of thinking (Leahy, 2001). Look at the following examples which show how far errors of thinking may apply to you as the worker.

1. Personalisation: 'Mental health has failed the client and I am to blame.'
2. Catastrophisation: 'The client feels suicidal and I cannot stand it.'
3. Labelling the client: 'This client is a nightmare.'
4. Labelling yourself: 'I am rubbish.'
5. Fortune telling: 'The client will never get better.'
6. Black and white thinking: 'Nothing works!'

Look back over the last week and the situations you have found yourself in with clients. How far did these categories apply in your work? Write down a few examples in your journal and then look at the following.

Alternative thoughts

You will remember from Chapter 2 we spoke about writing down alternative ways of looking at things. If any of the thinking errors above apply to you and your work, see how far the alternatives described below might help.

1. Personalisation: 'Clients may not get better for many reasons. You have helped others.'
2. Catastrophisation: 'Suicidal thoughts are common with people who are depressed. Nothing bad has happened yet and there are many things you can do to help. You can talk to others and arrange emergency care if needed.'
3. Labelling the client: 'The client is human and is suffering. She doesn't want to suffer, and the problems you are having with her are probably affecting her more than you. If you saw life through her eyes, your perspective may change.'

4. Labelling yourself: 'There are some people you can work with and some people you cannot. No one is perfect.'
5. Fortune telling: 'You do not know this. The reality is that many clients will improve even slightly and each person will have good and bad days. Look back over the past few weeks and see how their mood has fluctuated.'
6. Black and white thinking: 'Ask the client to look at his/her activity schedule from Chapter 5 and see how their mood fluctuates.'

Reflection

Over the next week reflect on your work with clients and identify some errors of thinking. Record them and then try to identify alternative thoughts. Make sure that you discuss these with your supervisor.

Exercise 6.2: Rules

Errors of thinking were part of the depression model that we discussed earlier. Rules and assumptions were also part of that model. Again, we can begin to apply some of the rules and assumptions to our work with clients. Look at the following rules and think how far these apply to you.

- I have to make everyone better.
- I must always be 100% perfect.
- Clients must appreciate everything I do for them.
- I should not feel bored when I am working with clients.
- I want to be liked by clients.
- I must not make a mistake.

If you have answered yes to any of them, make a record in your reflective journal with an example from practice. As with clients who are depressed, such rules can be a problem. As with errors of thinking, we try to 'reframe' these rules into guidance which feels more flexible. Challenging rules can be helpful in your work. In the list below you can see some of the questions that might be used in dealing with the rules above:

- Do all mental health workers achieve absolute perfection?
- Do we have to be perfect to make any progress?
- What are the reasons for applying such a high standard to yourself?
- Do other people think you should be perfect?
- Even if you are not perfect, what are the things you have done which have helped?

Think of someone who you are working with at the moment who has caused problems and apply some of the above challenges to yourself. How does this feel? Record your reflections and talk them through with your manager and/or supervisor.

Exercise 6.3: Core beliefs

In the earlier sections we talked about core beliefs. A useful metaphor for explaining this is to see core beliefs as having our 'buttons pushed'. Core beliefs are things which describe what we might feel vulnerable about. Think about the kinds of problems or clients that arouse strong feelings in you. What kind of client makes you feel depressed or angry or anxious? What is it about their communication style that bothers you?

Exercise 6.4: Coping strategies

We have rules and assumptions and we have ways of coping. The Four Aspects Model refers to behaviour. Behaviour in this sense describes how someone copes. If a client is making us feel vulnerable we may cope in different ways. If clients make us feel angry or helpless, we may switch off emotionally when we are with them.

When you have worked with a client who has presented you with difficulties how do you cope? Describe specifically what you do. How useful or not useful is it?

Exercise 6.5: The problem with empathy

We may feel that some clients' core beliefs and vulnerabilities are the same as ours. In relation to their likes, dislikes and their personality they may be very similar to us. We may begin to respond to them as if they are friends. Part of this might be driven by the need to be approved of by clients. We naturally want to make clients feel good but this can be at the expense of avoiding areas of difficulty through a fear of conflict. How far does any of this apply to you? Write down some examples. If it does not apply to you, give the reasons why but then proceed to the next exercise.

Exercise 6.6: Your own empathy

There can also be a problem with a lack of empathy. In many health and social care settings there is an emphasis on being professional. While this is understandable, there may be problems in having boundaries which are too rigid. For example, a 'professional' relationship can come across as dispassionate. This may lead the client to feel that their suffering is not acknowledged and may lead them to believe that they cannot engage with the worker.

What problems could you foresee with yourself?

Reflection

It is likely that this chapter has given you much food for thought. You may have found that Exercises 6.5 and 6.6 did not apply to you and you have been able to manage the need to be empathic while at the same time maintaining boundaries. If this is the case then reflect on how you have managed this. What is it that you did right? With the other areas, make sure that you use one of your supervision sessions to discuss them with your supervisor, as this is an issue which is crucial in relation to your work. Look back on the exercises from this section and discuss them. Also review the contents of your reflective journal and consider how far any problems that you experienced were due to 'errors of thinking'. Make a note of any previous situations and consider what you might do to begin to change the pattern.

Conclusion

Good mental health often focuses on the so-called work/life balance. There will of course be times when events from our personal lives will affect our work. In such circumstances it is important to check whether or not you are ok enough to be at work. Not doing this might tap into the rule of 'I should be able to tolerate this, I work in mental health'.

This section has in effect involved practising CBT skills on yourself. It is to be hoped that the areas that you have covered in this section will be of use for many years to come.

References

Leahy R (2001) *Overcoming Resistance in Cognitive Therapy.* New York: Guilford.

Wilde McCormick E (2008) *Change for the Better* (3rd edition). London: SAGE Publications.

Chapter 7: Maintaining progress

Learning outcomes

By the end of this section you will know how to:

- develop a plan to continue developing skills.
- identify triggers and warning signs for depression.
- identify a plan for maintaining health.

QCF units

Health and Social Care Diploma Level 3

- Unit CMH 301: Understand mental well-being and mental health promotion. Learning outcomes 1and 2.

This final section looks at how workers can encourage clients to continue to practise their skills to maintain their progress when they are about to leave your service. We will look at how to develop a relapse prevention plan. By this stage the client should be able to use the skills previously taught and has hopefully been able to demonstrate some progress.

Relapse in depression

As we have stated in Chapter 1, relapse in depression will always be a possibility. It is therefore important for the worker to set aside time to address these potential issues with the client. The goal of any work with a client is to ensure that they are able to use the skills that they have learnt independently for their own benefit.

Continuing the work they have started

Clients by this stage may have invested a great deal into their recovery and it is important to emphasise that continuing this work is crucial to their continued well-being. Many clients may by this stage view themselves as well, and might think that they do not need to continue to use their new-found skills. This can be a problem as a full recovery from depression requires ongoing practice in the skills of CBT.

One way of addressing this issue is to ensure that you discuss with the client how they can continue their sessions on their own in the future. It is important to be sensitive to the needs of the client at this stage as there needs to be a balance between ensuring the client is aware of continuing to address their problems but at the same time not minimising achievements that they have already made. An example of how you might start the conversation may go like this:

Worker: *'Shall we think about how you might continue the work you have started here, so that you can use these skills and techniques to keep yourself well in the future?'*

Client: *'Do I need to do that? I am well now.'*

Worker: *'I understand that you now feel better and you have achieved a great deal and just want to get on with your life, but depression does have a high rate of relapse and it would be really helpful if you could continue to use what you have learned. Shall we look at how you might do that?'*

Client: *'Ok, yes, I don't want to get unwell again in the future.'*

Exercise 7.1: Relapse prevention – continuing practice

Go through Handout 7.1 with the client and think about how they might begin to schedule time in their week to continue to work on keeping well.

Exercise 7.2: Planning skills

When you have completed Exercise 7.1 you will need to 'break down' each section and develop a plan for each of the areas. As we have done in previous exercises, practise this on yourself. Complete a plan for yourself using Handout 7.2 as a guide. This handout names some of the key skills we have already spoken about.

When you complete this handout for yourself, think about the third column. What are the outcomes you would look for from using the skills? If you become skilled in using the Four Aspects Model, think about how this could help. If you are clear about what activities give you a sense of pleasure and/or mastery, think about how this might help? Here is an example of this.

Situation or event	Skills	Outcome
Argument with family.	Look at the Four Aspects Model, identify any errors of thinking and core beliefs. Challenge and reframe thoughts. Identify avoidance behaviour and challenge these.	Helped thinking about it differently. Recognised I was able to be assertive and, rather than isolating myself, I could go and talk to a friend.

Once you have completed this and you are happy with it, then you can action the plan over the following week. Be sure to note down the outcomes including any reasons why you didn't get to do the practice.

Exercise 7.3: Planning skills practice

Now use Handout 7.3 with one of your clients. When completing it, try to ensure that you cover most if not all of the skills that have been learned over the period that you have worked with them.

Reflection

You may notice, as in your own practice, that there are times when your client didn't stick to the plan – they may say things such as they 'forgot', or 'there wasn't enough time', or 'I couldn't be bothered, I was too tired or I didn't need to'. This kind of scenario can happen. If it does, make a note of this in your journal and talk about this with your supervisor or manager. Think about some of the possible barriers. It may be helpful here to refer back to the previous chapter and remember the importance of not coming across as critical or judgemental. As we mentioned earlier, it is important to gently emphasise the need to continue to practise.

Identifying triggers and coping with setbacks

In this section, you as the worker are supporting the client to identify possible trigger situations that may occur in the future that they may be vulnerable to. These trigger situations are those events or experiences that may result in mood lowering in the first instance and have the potential to trigger a relapse in the future. Many clients will possibly already be aware of certain situations that may trip them up but it is useful to plan for these anyway.

Exercise 7.4: Identifying triggers

As the worker, think about your own life experiences and those that may have an impact on how you feel. Think about your triggers. Can you identify any scenarios or situations that may make you feel anxious, angry or sad, in particular those events that may stay on your mind for a while? Look at the table below as an example. Now complete Handout 7.4 and list some of your triggers, focusing on the type of thoughts, emotions and behaviours you may have.

Situation or event	Thoughts	Emotions	Behaviours	Consequences
Had an argument with a family member about the dog.	It's my fault. I should not be so selfish. Why didn't I just take him out.	Sadness. Anger. Guilt.	Sit and cry. Ruminate about it. Isolate myself.	Mood becomes lower and thinking will become more negative.

Reflection

Having completed this exercise you should have a list of scenarios that may potentially trigger a change in mood. When completing this with the client, focus on those triggers that may lower their mood and therefore become the start of a cycle of depressed thinking. It may be helpful to review some of the information on the vicious circle nature of depression from Chapter 3. Helping the client to identify how what they have learned can help with these situations can be incredibly helpful. Being aware of these triggers and potentially how you can manage them means that they are already prepared for them. Emphasising that negative thinking will only lead to worsening of mood reinforces the vicious circle of depression. Make a note of some of these factors and share them with your supervisor or manager.

Identifying signs and symptoms of relapse

We discussed in Chapter 2 that once someone has experienced depression, the likelihood of them relapsing in the future can be quite high. In the previous section we discussed some of the trigger situations which may lead to clients becoming depressed again. It will be important that each client is aware of their own individual signs and symptoms of relapse. If clients are aware of these then the likelihood of being able to intervene when they notice them is greater. Often depression creeps up on us and there is a pattern; mood becoming lower, thinking becoming more negative and then engaging in unhelpful coping strategies. A signs and symptoms checklist can be developed with the client that they can keep and refer to when needed.

Exercise 7.5: Signs and symptoms of relapse

Make a list of all the signs and symptoms that different people may notice if they are becoming depressed. You will have already learned some of these from the previous chapters in the book and your experience of working with different clients. You may also be aware of signs and symptoms from your own personal experience.

As the worker, you will now be more familiar with their particular problems with depression and can assist the client in developing their own signs and symptoms list. An example of how you might address this with your client is given below.

Worker: *'It may be helpful to have a think about what might happen if you were to become unwell again. If we can learn to recognise our own signs and symptoms of relapse it means that we can perhaps act much sooner and stop the illness developing further.'*

Client: *'OK.'*

Worker: *'So what would be the things that tell you that you are starting to become unwell again? We can then write them onto the template.'*

As you and the client identify these signs and symptoms write them on Handout 7.5. If the client struggles with this you can ask them to get family or friends to help by pointing out what they noticed, or refer back to the DSM-V criteria for depression to remind them.

Exercise 7.6: Developing an action plan

Once the client has been able to identify some of their own personal signs and symptoms of relapse, it can then be helpful to look at an action plan as to how they may manage these once they appear. Managing these symptoms may require using the skills previously taught in this manual or it may mean seeking help from others. Again, it can be helpful for the client to think about these prior to them occurring so that they are more prepared. Look at the following dialogue.

Worker: *'Ok, well done. You now have a list of some of your relapse symptoms which may make it easier to spot them if they occur.'*

Client: *'Yeah. Actually it helps to remember that you do not just wake up with depression, but that it starts gradually and develops.'*

Worker: *'Yes that's true, and if you can spot the symptoms before depression really takes hold then you may be able to prevent it from getting worse.*

Client: *'That would be good.'*

Worker: *'I agree. So now we have our list of symptoms, perhaps we can think about what you can do if you notice them appearing.'*

Once the client has a good understanding of how early action can prevent depression from really taking hold then you can plan what skills or strategies you may use. An example is given below. Develop an action plan with the client using Handout 7.6.

Example action plan	
Signs and symptoms of relapse	**Actions**
Feeling tired and going to bed in the day.	Try not going to bed and doing a small activity instead that will give a degree of mastery or pleasure. Am I doing too much and need to cut back a bit?
Starting to feel negative and self-critical.	Use vicious circle model to identify unhelpful thoughts. Am I using a thinking error? Can I challenge my thought and come up with a more balanced alternative? Make appointment with GP.
Not wanting to go out and meet with friends.	Identify thoughts associated with this and look to challenge these thoughts. Remember the first thing we give up on when we feel depressed is activities for ourselves. Try not to avoid going out and be compassionate to self.

Improving the way you feel about yourself

As we will know by now, people with depression often think very negatively about themselves and have low self-esteem. Even after recovering from depression some of these thoughts can remain, and if negative thinking was to take hold again this could then lead to further episodes of depression. It is therefore important that the client takes some time to look after themselves, even when feeling better. A useful strategy to complete when well is to develop a list of positive qualities. We already know from our knowledge about negative automatic thoughts that when our mood becomes low we filter out all positive and pleasant things going on around us. The thinking error of filtering from the list in Chapter 4 (p33) can be a helpful reminder of how we discount positive qualities. Revisiting activities of mastery and pleasure from Chapter 5 will also help.

Exercise 7.7: Your positive qualities

Develop a list of your own positive qualities using Handout 7.7. You can also ask friends and family what they think are good qualities that you as a person have, for example: kind, caring, a good cook.

The idea is to obtain a good list of all the positive qualities that you have and then monitor on a regular basis when these qualities occur. This can then act as a record which clients can refer back to when they notice that their mood is becoming low or that they are beginning to think negatively about themselves.

Exercise 7.8: The client's positive qualities

Now give the client a copy of Handout 7.8 and ask them to develop a list of their positive qualities. As the worker, you can help them identify these qualities. They can then take the form away with them and ask family and friends who they trust. Note that you are only asking the client to list positive qualities.

Exercise 7.9: Examples

Once the client has compiled their list of positive qualities then the next step is to look at days when they demonstrate this positive quality. This can be quite a difficult task for clients even when well. Below is an example of how you might record this. Ask them to fill out Handout 7.9 when particular examples of their positive qualities occur.

Example

Positive quality	Example
1. Good at organising.	1. Organised a night out with friends next week.
2. Fun to be with.	2. Played games with kids at tea time. Had a good laugh.
3. Caring towards others.	3. Had a chat with a friend who is having a tough time. He thanked me for being there.

Reflection

These records can be helpful for clients if they notice that their mood is dropping and they are starting to think negatively. At times, if their mood is low they may need to use some of the activities linked with mastery and pleasure from Chapter 5 and the thinking errors sheet from Chapter 3. This will ensure that they keep focused on doing what works as well as challenging their thinking.

At this stage it may help to look at some of the comments made about goals in Chapter 1. Exercise 1.5 looks at setting goals, however, goals need to be underpinned by values. Values are the kinds of things which make life worth living, they are the principles and standards that determine the degree of worth or merit of an object or act to that particular person (Hayes *et al*, 2011). In his work on acceptance and commitment therapy, Steven Hayes noted that Martin Luther King Jr. didn't achieve any of his goals but his life was seen as a success because he lived according to his values. In this sense a life lived according to what is important or of value will be the best help in living a life where episodes of low mood or depression can be managed effectively.

What to do in the event of relapse

Given everything that we have spoken about in this chapter, it is important to take into account the worst-case scenario for clients with depression. As we mentioned at the start of this chapter the possibility of relapse is high for clients who have experienced more than one episode of depression. For many, much more in-depth psychotherapy is going to be necessary and it is important that they are able to access help if needed. It can also be helpful for family and friends of the client to know how to access help if required. It is important that as a worker we ensure that clients are fully aware of what support is available to them should they need it. It will therefore be helpful to develop an 'action card'.

As a worker it will be important to consider the issue of relapse. Many clients might feel ashamed that they have relapsed and see it as some flaw within themselves, that perhaps they have not done enough practice or perhaps they deserved it in some way. Again, this thinking becomes the background to depression and we begin to filter information around us in a particularly negative way.

Exercise 7.9: Action card

Work with the client in developing an action card. As the worker, see if you can find out all the services available to someone who may be currently depressed and need support. Your manager, supervisor or other members of the team you work in may be able to help. These may be voluntary agencies and support groups or healthcare related services. It can be very helpful to be prepared with this information when assisting a client to develop an action card as you are likely to be more aware of services available. Ensure that you have up-to-date contact telephone numbers and opening hours. Information contained on the action card relates to simple steps that a client can take when depressed and helps them to access support when required. It is important that they recognise if they are a risk to themselves then they will need to seek professional help as soon as possible. An example of this is given in Handout 7.9.

Reflection

The action card can be tailored to your work area and location depending on what services you have available in your area. Ensure that you discuss them or any other similar tools that you may have in your team with your supervisor or manager.

Conclusion

The pathway in this manual looks at the pathway of a client at the point of entering your service and leaving your service. We hope that this has helped you with an understanding of the framework and tools of cognitive behavioural therapy. The manual is not a substitute for the therapy itself. If you have worked with people using these techniques and they do not seem to have worked, think about re-referral to workers with more formal training in CBT. As we suggested in the previous exercise, this will mean that it will be important for you to know what services exist in your area.

As a final note, it needs to be emphasised that this book is not a substitute for substantive psychotherapy training. If in the course of working through this manual you think that you would like to work as a CBT therapist, the British Association for Behavioural and Cognitive Psychotherapies (http://www.babcp.com/Default.aspx) will give details of further training.

We wish you luck.

References

Hayes SC, Strosahl KD & Wilson KG (2011) *Acceptance and Commitment Therapy: The process and practice of mindful change* (2nd edition). New York: Guilford Press.

Handout 7.1

Exercise 7.1: Relapse prevention – continuing practice

Most people recovering from depression may face some difficult or unpleasant situations or events in the months after their treatment. To avoid the symptoms of depression returning and to help you cope with difficulties and setbacks, it is important that you continue to practise the skills you have learned. There are five main areas to work on:

1. Putting your skills into practice.
2. Identifying triggers and coping with setbacks.
3. Improving how you feel about yourself.
4. Understanding your signs and symptoms of relapse.
5. What to do in the event of relapse.

During your treatment for depression you may have found that you have had access to different types of support. It is assumed that if you are reading this handout that you have been working with someone who has helped you learn a number of skills and techniques from cognitive behaviour therapy. You may have met with them on a regular basis and have found it helpful to talk about the problems you are having. Unfortunately, when you become well this support will come to an end and you may find it difficult to find the time to put your skills into practice.

1. Putting skills into practice

It is more helpful to do a little bit of practice regularly rather than set aside large chunks of time each week. You will also need a space where you can focus on this practice without being interrupted by telephone calls or partners and children. By continuing this practice on a regular basis you are more likely to have confidence in the skills when you do need to use them. It can be helpful to review your practice notes and look at what helped the most, then you can review your week and identify any areas of concern where it may be helpful to use the skills learned.

2. Identifying triggers and coping with setbacks

When you have experienced depression, it can be very easy to fall back into unhelpful habits and ways of thinking. Identifying stressful situations or events where you are likely to experience difficulty is essential in keeping well. If you are able to identify these trigger situations then you can prepare for them. Review your week and next few months for any situations or events that may potentially trip you up. For some people this can include things like an argument with someone, being asked to do too much at work, or even visiting family members who know you have been unwell. It can be helpful to think about what you can do that may help you cope in this situation? What has helped in the past when these things happened? Is there anything you can do next time this happens?

Handout 7.1 (continued)

3. Improving how you feel about yourself

You will have been aware that when depressed our confidence and self-esteem suffers. You will most probably have done some work around this if you have been working with someone. This is because low self-esteem helps maintain depression and it is therefore important that you continue to address it as part of your recovery and beyond. One way of addressing this is to keep a daily diary or log of the times when you have evidence that you have acted against a negative belief. An example of this may be that your negative view of your self is that 'I am a failure'. Keeping a log of times when things have gone well for you despite this belief can be a helpful way of improving low self-esteem. Continuing to engage in activities that give you a sense of mastery or pleasure is also important in improving confidence and low self-esteem. Reflecting on how you did and addressing any issues straight away will make it less likely that you will fall into unhealthy patterns that may start to water the seeds of depression.

4. Identifying signs and symptoms of relapse

It is important that you are aware of your own signs and symptoms of relapse and know what you can do when you notice these so that you can intervene and 'nip it in the bud' before it becomes too much of a problem. Developing a signs and symptoms checklist can be important to remind you of these and perhaps what action you can take. Enlisting the support of loved ones and friends can also be helpful and ensuring that they are also aware of these relapse signs. This will ensure that 1) people do not overreact and 2) they are aware of what would be helpful at that time. You can also give your GP a copy of your plan too.

5. What to do in the event of relapse

It is important to have a plan of 'what to do' if you start to recognise that you are becoming unwell again. Having a plan of what to do and who to contact at these times can take some of the stress out of the situation. It can also be helpful for family members and friends to be aware of what to do as this can be a worrying time for everyone. Ensure that you have appropriate contact numbers for those who may be able to help and can offer support.

Handout 7.2

Exercise 7.2: Planning skills

Day	Skills to practise	Outcome
Monday	Use the Four Aspects Model to map out an event. Read through the thinking errors sheet and identify any in the thoughts section. Can you reframe these thoughts into something more helpful?	
Tuesday	Monitor activities during the day and rate them for pleasure and achievement.	

Handout 7.3

Exercise 7.3: Planning skills practice

Day	Skills to practise	Outcome
Monday		
Tuesday		
Wednesday		
Thursday		
Friday		
Saturday		
Sunday		

Handout 7.4

Exercise 7.4: Identifying triggers

Situation or event	Thoughts	Emotions	Behaviours	Consequences

Handout 7.5

Exercise 7.5: Signs and symptoms of relapse

Handout 7.6

Exercise 7.6: Developing an action plan

Sign or symptom of relapse	Actions

Handout 7.7

Exercise 7.7: Your positive qualities

Positive qualities

Handout 7.8

Exercise 7.8: The client's positive qualities

Positive qualities

Handout 7.9

Exercise 7.9: Examples

Day	Positive quality	Example
Monday		
Tuesday		
Wednesday		
Thursday		
Friday		
Saturday		
Sunday		

Handout 7.9

Exercise 7.9: Action card

Relapse action card for ....

- Acknowledge that you are depressed and need help.
- Try as best you can to use the skills and techniques learned for helping with depression.
- Contact your GP and make an appointment. Your medication may need reviewing
  [GP telephone number and opening hours and out of hours GP service]
  111 [non-emergency medical help]
- Contact a friend/colleague/family member or professional you trust to support you at this time.
  [Name of supporter or professional including telephone number]
- Try not to isolate yourself.
- Seek professional help from mental health services.
- IF IT BECOMES WORSE and you are at risk of hurting yourself then access the out of hours GP, Samaritans or other services in your area.
  [e.g. Samaritans 0845 7909090]